TEACHING
STUDENTS
WITH
LEARNING
DISABILITIES

STRATEGIES FOR SUCCESS

TEACHING STUDENTS WITH LEARNING DISABILITIES

STRATEGIES FOR SUCCESS

Karen A. Waldron, Ph.D.
Associate Professor
Department of Education
Trinity University
San Antonio, Texas

SINGULAR PUBLISHING GROUP, INC.
San Diego, California

Singular Publishing Group, Inc.
4284 41st Street
San Diego, California 92105-1197

Waldron, Karen A., 1945-
    Teaching students with learning disabilities: strategies for success /
    Karen A. Waldron.
        p.   cm.
    Includes bibliographical references and index.
    ISBN 1-879105-40-3
    1. Learning disabled children—Education—United States.
2. Classroom management—United States.   3. Parent-teacher relationships—
United States.   I. Title.
LC4704.W33   1992
371.9'043'0973—dc20   91-42271
                                                       CIP

Typeset by House Graphics
Typeset in 11/13 Garamond
Printed by McNaughton & Gunn
Cover clock artwork used with permission, Winston School, San Antonio, Texas

Printed in the United States of America

Contents

Dedication

To Michael J. Kutchins, my wonderful husband and friend, and to my delightful family of sons, James and Matt Waldron, Jack and Jeff Ko, each of whose lives has been touched by caring teachers.

Acknowledgments

Writing a book is an effort which goes far beyond the capabilities of any individual. The experiences, observations, and expertise of educators on the "firing lines" daily are the fabric for understanding the present and for formulating the future. There have been fine professionals who have dedicated time beyond their schedules to help in the publication of this book.

So many thanks for their wonderful support go to:

The Department of Education, fine colleagues and friends at Trinity University, and the field-based program emphasizing that teaching matters, and that the student is the reason we are here;

The students at Trinity: young, bright, and proof that there are teachers who care;

The many teachers, from New York to Texas, who have let me tell their story;

Sammie Perry, and the incredible teachers and staff at Carrollton-Farmers Branch ISD, Texas, for their creativity and ability to forge new directions in educations for the handicapped;

Cha Karulak and the fine teachers and staff at Winston School, San Antonio, Texas, for realizing that "special" schools must be special, and providing the expertise that has underscored so many suggestions in this text;

Nancy Ellis, Resource Teacher, Alamo Heights ISD, San Antonio, Texas, whose planning, organization, but mostly, caring, has touched the lives of so many children;

Bernie Dailey, Maxine Smith, and Virginia Zoncki-Bunker and the fine teachers and staff in St. Paul, Minnesota, for the philosophy "We just try to do what's best for the children";

Lisa Coriell Davis, a former student of whom anyone could be proud, but especially, a woman of vision and caring;

Michael Kutchins, whose knowledge of computers and communications has made this text possible; and

Michael Bender, a wonderful editor, who instilled enjoyment and reflection into the process of writing this book.

Preface

Barbara Myers has finally reached her limit. While she has taught students with learning disabilities for 6 years and has enjoyed the excitement of students learning to read and students who are language delayed expressing themselves better, things have certainly changed. Most noticeably the children are different. While Barbara used to concentrate on teaching word-attack skills or arithmetic problem-solving, she now spends most of her time managing behaviors. These days, many of her students seem incapable of attending to any academic task for more than a few minutes. They rarely control their impulses, and yell across the classroom or leave their seats at will. As Barbara notes, "I'm seeing more and more evidence of the social craziness I read about in the newspapers. Five years ago, most of my students came to school with a night's sleep and breakfast, and the majority even did their homework. Now we're not supposed to expect anything. I have students sleeping in class, stealing money for lunch, and I've been advised not to give homework since it won't be done anyway. This year I have the first of my 'crack' kids. One of them hits his classmates constantly and the other just starts screaming when he can't get his way. Yet, the primary diagnosis for both is 'learning disabled' and I'm supposed to change their behaviors as well as teach them academics. I'm not sure what 'learning disabilities' means any more because of the extent of behavioral problems in each of my classes."

But the learning problems certainly are there too. The majority of children Barbara sees have difficulties in reading and other language areas, as well as in math, especially when solving word problems or performing basic computation. During her first period class alone, Barbara's real task is to teach Jane and Marcos phonics, especially consonant blends and diagraphs; to work with Heather on reading comprehension for main ideas; to teach Juan and Kevin arithmetic problem-solving, although at two vastly different grade levels; to improve Jake's handwriting; to expand

Linda's expressive vocabulary and Carlos' verbal syntax; and to work with Cathy, severely below her peers in all areas.

Because scheduling is almost more difficult than teaching, Barbara finds that she cannot easily combine students with similar learning problems or achievement levels in the same class. It is not unusual to be instructing students in four or five different need areas and at achievement levels that may vary by years. While she is currently trying to expand the blocks of time students spend in her class, she frequently only has children 30 or 40 minutes a day, and even they arrive at different intervals, interrupting others as they enter the room.

Understandably, all of this has affected Barbara's attitude toward her job. "I used to like to come to work, but now I'm really burned out. The structure is terrible, and when you add disruptive student behaviors and parents who don't seem to care, I don't see how any of us can win. The kids seem to have picked up my sense of failure and we've lost any fun or excitement in the room. I've taught 'dyslexics' and 'dysgraphics' for years, but I feel like I've developed 'dysfunctionitis.' What can I do?"

This book will focus on specific ways to help Barbara—and you—regain control of learning and behavior in the classroom, for without this control it is likely that you both will leave teaching and more good teachers will be lost by the children. Discussion will emphasize how educators in resource class-rooms, Content Mastery units, and regular education settings can teach students with learning disabilities and enjoy the process. While much has been written on the theoretical aspects of exceptional learners, this book is practical in its intent. It is based on the reality that students are different today, posing far more difficult problems than ever before, and that educators need a variety of specific strategies to be successful. The many suggestions in this book are based on best practices research, but especially from daily experiences of teachers on the "firing lines." None of the strategies cost money, underscor-ing the belief that what we do in the classroom is more important than what we spend.

A series of concerns to practitioners will be explored: How can teachers create a positive atmosphere but still take charge? How can student records be more useful in daily work? Can students become motivated, leaving lethargy behind and actively participating in classroom learning? What discipline systems really work so that the teacher can more easily direct student behaviors? How can collaborative systems between regular and special education be more effective so that educators share information and support children? How can teachers organize their classrooms so that students will begin and complete their work more independently? Are there ways that interactions with parents can be more meaningful, inviting them to work closely with the school?

To deal with some of the academic and behavioral problems in school today, it is important to first understand their nature. Discussion will explore a re-design of the classroom, putting teachers back in charge of learning in the midst of an environment where both they and students can experience success. This book is about positive teaching and feeling positively about the children we teach.

Chapter 1

MEETING A DIVERSITY OF NEEDS

Unfortunately, many children with learning disabilities tend to be drop-outs or cast-offs from a system where there has been a mismatch. By definition, these students have not integrated information at the same rate or to the same degree as the "non-disabled." Since they have not learned in the way most teachers instruct, they have been designated as the problem.

Yet most of these children possess learning *differences*, not disabilities, and the fault may actually lie within inflexible classroom methods, not within the child. The needs of students with disabilities are the same as any child's: to learn to read, write, compute, and have happy, independent, and productive lives. However, because educators and related staff are limited in awareness of successful ways to work with children with learning differences, these critical goals are threatened. An alternative system has been produced with the expectation that it will be more responsive to differences.

The folly of this separate system derives from its basic premise that all students with learning disabilities are alike and can be served in the same way. Nothing is further from the truth. "Learning disabilities" (note the plural) are a hodgepodge of areas where children are not performing at expectancy levels. The discipline was created in an attempt to serve the many children who did not fit into the previous categorical molds, but who were experiencing school-related problems (Kirk, 1963). Broad terms such as "learning disabilities" were never intended to provide a diagnosis of a problem, but only to indicate the general direction for subsequent funding and programming. It is imperative to look within the category for the specific problem preventing or inhibiting learning and not to be overwhelmed or misdirected by a name.

A mainstream classroom teacher was told by assessment personnel at the beginning of the year that one of her students, a 9-year-old girl, was "dyslexic." Although the student attended a resource class for 50 minutes each day during that year, she received her primary instruction in the regular classroom. When the spring meeting was held to review her progress, the staff was disheartened to learn that she had not only shown poor progress in reading, but that her skills were actually lower than when the year began. Her regular classroom teacher shrugged and responded, "What do you expect? She's dyslexic." If the teacher had been given more specific information, such as the student's having few sight words in her reading vocabulary, based on a poor visual memory, the teacher could have concentrated on the specific problem instead of being threatened by a broad clinical diagnosis.

A person labeled "learning disabled" may demonstrate any of a variety of problems, as demonstrated in Figures 1-1, 1-2, and 1-3. An examination of the possibilities for reading dysfunction alone indicates that general categories will not work for individual students. For example, some students with visual-spatial problems will experience difficulty with left-right directionality in reading, while others with language disorders may have problems with auditory discrimination of similar sounds, debilitating phonics use. Others may have cognitive processing disorders in categorizing information, while some will categorize properly but have problems with sequential memory. Language disorders, whether in receiving, processing, or expressing information, certainly can affect reading comprehension and subsequent written expression. The difficulty occurs when these students are grouped together as if their learning strengths and problems are all the same and can be overcome by identical instructional methods. If a leg is broken, it will not help to set an arm. It is important to teach to students' needs if their skills are to improve.

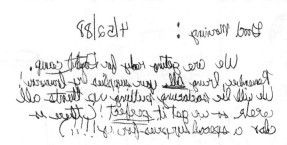

Copied from the blackboard at school, the message should read:

4/24/88

Good Morning:

We are getting ready for overnight camp. Remember, bring _all_ your supplies by tomorrow. We will be practicing putting up tents all week so we get it _perfect!_ (There is also a special prize for you!!!!)

Figure 1-1. Mirror-writing of a child with visual-perceptual problems. Reprinted with permission, Winston School, San Antonio, Texas.

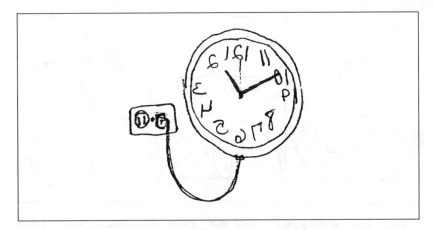

Figure 1-2. Clock drawn by child with visual-perceptual problems. Reprinted with permission, Winston School, San Antonio, Texas.

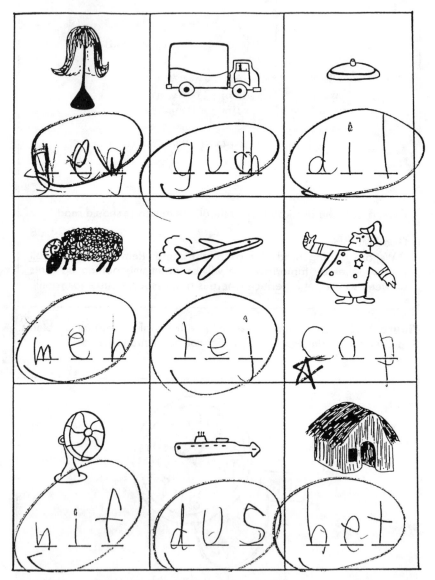

Figure 1-3. Writing of a child with visual- and auditory-perception problems. Reprinted with the permission of Educators Publishing Service, Cambridge, Massachusetts, and the Winston School, San Antonio, Texas.

ATTENTION DEFICIT HYPERACTIVITY DISORDER

Unfortunately, along with academic and behavioral problems, children with learning differences often experience Attention Deficit Hyperactivity Disorder (ADHD) (American Psychiatric Association, 1987). These problems with concentration and attention often have seemed to be Nature's cruel overlay on students who are already experiencing lack of school success. If students are having difficulty tracking a line of print or aligning numbers in arithmetic computation, the teaching-learning situation is worsened a hundredfold when they cannot stay in their seats or attend to the text on their desk. Children with ADHD often have a short attention span, sometimes no more than a few minutes. Many times they are distracted by any sound or movement, lessening their concentration in a typical busy classroom. They tend to be frustrated easily, for example, tearing up their worksheet if they are experiencing problems or refusing to attempt a new task if it looks difficult. The hyperactivity element is one that most teachers dread: The students have a "physical motor" which is difficult to stop and causes them to leave their desks often, climb on their seats, and have difficulty staying seated for any length of time. As experts such as Hewett (1968) note, it is difficult for students to learn a task if they are not paying attention.

Actually, ADHD children *are* paying attention. But they are paying attention to the wrong thing. As part of their distractibility, they are focusing as much on the sound of the heater or other students talking as on the teacher giving directions. They may be masters at selecting bits of visual or auditory data without integrating the whole. A school psychologist noted how a young, visually distractible student once interrupted an item during intelligence testing to comment on the psychologist's contact lenses. The student had known the psychologist only minutes, but had picked out that fine detail; others had known her for years, but never realized she wore contact lenses.

DIRECTIVE TEACHERS

Because of the behavioral and academic problems in Barbara's classroom, one message is very clear: Barbara has a need to take charge (not necessarily to "take *control*"). When teach-ers take charge, they create situations where students learn in a variety of ways, sometimes directed by the teacher's learning goals and sometimes by students' interests. Teachers in charge, or "Directive Teachers," need to feel that they understand student learning problems thoroughly, are knowledgeable in methods of remediation and compensation, and can aptly manage student behaviors. These teachers do not always need to be "front and center" in a classroom or to direct all learning that takes place, but they do need to have students respond positively to them and to demonstrate behaviors conducive to learning, such as staying in seats, listening, following directions, speaking only when appropriate, and actively participating in a friendly, nonhostile way to assignments and activities. (These needs are so basic that they are hardly ones for which teachers, or anyone, should have to ask. Yet many teachers today tend to feel that students are doing them a favor by being respectful or nonhostile in any way.)

Directive Teachers realize that, while much learning takes place outside structured lessons, often students do need to be guided toward academic areas of need, such as reading, which students might not choose independently because of a history of difficulty and subsequent lack of motivation. For a number of years, "Carson School," a private "open school" allowed students a totally free choice selection of daily instructional activities in which to participate. Although ungraded, the school included students from 5 through 14 years of age, approximately kin-dergarten to eighth grade, was designed and supported by an in-novative university education department, and primarily included children of liberal community members and university faculty. While many preschools enjoy a free-flowing Piagetian-based curriculum and allow student choice of activities, Carson School followed the "free-choice" model for all ages of students. With the philosophy that students are most motivated when they have selected their tasks, students were permitted to take charge of their own learning, with teachers present only as facilitators. If children were particularly motivated to study science or art, they involved themselves in learning centers, studios, and laboratories for months and often years, to the exclusion of areas of lesser interest. While some students further developed a sense of curiosity and broadness because of stimulating experiences across an array of areas, they were a distinct minority. Carson School became the birthplace of specialists, of future scientists who could not perform the most basic of mathematical operations, of artists who could not read because they were allowed to exclusively pursue areas of interest and avoided those that were more difficult, or required sustained effort. Carson School failed and is now closed. Its positive lesson is that with active involvement in a highly stimulating environment students will become excited about learning and want to pursue their interests. Its negative lesson is that students can never fully "take charge" of their own learning, that they must be directed through activities and exercises that will expose them to an array of academics and support them in areas of difficulty.

It is of no surprise that Carson School's greatest failure was in not creating proficient readers and writers, and that the largest numbers of students who chose not to study reading or writing entered Carson School with learning problems. "Why do it if it hurts?" might have been asked by many of these children. Their parents reported that as time progressed and the students were as young as 8 or 9 years of age, they would avoid reading and writing tasks, especially when they were around their neighborhood peers, through fear of embarrassment at deficient skills. A type of progressive dyslexia was actually cultivated by the environment.

A Directive Teacher would use the stimulating environment of Carson School as a basis for encouraging student exploration of a variety of areas. Children would be required to spend a designated amount of time daily in each content area, but with activities and materials at individualized levels. Students would be provided choices, but in ways that are appropriate to their age and learning style. For example, a student could select a preferred book to reinforce phonics skills from texts or select the method of initiating a writing assignment such as taping or dictating it to a classmate. But the student would not have the choice of doing phonics versus completing the writing assignment. Directive Teachers provide activities while allowing selection of motivational supports.

CONTROLLING TEACHERS

In contrast, "Controlling Teachers" also direct learning, but select reinforcement for students and provide a more "front-and-center" appearance. Controlling Teachers tend to lecture more and to provide fewer choices for students. More traditional in their approach, they tend to rely less on learning centers and cooperative interactions between students, and to concentrate on similar reinforcement for all students, often through rote paperwork.

Controlling Teachers often do not understand that learning problems can be dramatically different and that dissimilar needs rarely can be met through similar instruction. They have forgotten that the student, not the teacher, is the most important person in the classroom, and that to meet individual needs the educators and related staff must use differentiated instruction, varied academic practice, and behavioral reinforcements. Ironically, it is rare that the Controlling Teacher actually has the desired academic or behavioral control of the classroom.

While it would be simplistic to say that there is always a cause-effect relationship between degree of control and teacher attitude, it is common that those teachers who feel most positive about themselves as people, about teaching as a profession, and about children in general tend to be more directive than controlling in their teaching styles.

A poignant episode occurred several years ago at a local elementary school when parents were taking their children to the first day of kindergarten. Although many of the children were veterans of nursery school, they were understandably nervous at their first venture into a public elementary school. This nervousness was mixed with happiness and excitement at now being among the "big kids" in the neighborhood, surely a rite of passage. The children in the class were similarly ambivalent in their feelings, as a few shooed their parents away, while most clung warily. The parents were delighted to see how a caring teacher was already preparing for an exciting first day. She met them at the door and greeted parents, listening to their concerns while she kept a caring arm around a young shoulder. She led each child to a cheery desk covered with the student's name, a piece of candy, and a small present—pencils and crayons. The children adjusted very quickly and began to ignore their parents in favor of the engaging new situation. As these parents left, they were taken with the bright welcoming atmosphere in a classroom that did not even have windows. It was clearly the teacher's attitude toward the children and school that made all of them feel so positive.

As the parents left the building, they walked past the main entrance where they were startled by shouting and a small gathering of students. In the center of the commotion was a student large enough to be a fifth grader, who was screaming that he would not go inside the school building and that his very upset mother, standing nearby, could not make him. He used numerous profanities as he described how much he hated school, and most unlikely for a boy his age, cried openly. Understandably, his mother seemed bewildered as to what to do or say, and she quietly just asked him to go to his classroom. He refused and continued to cry.

The contrast was marked between the positive atmosphere of the kindergarten classroom and this negative scene. What could have happened to this young man in 5 or 6 years that would have impacted his feelings so negatively? His mother did not seem like an awful person, and his venom had been directed completely toward the school, not toward her or other factors, indicating that the school did seem to be the locus of the problem. Would he have been as resistant if many of his teachers had been as positive toward him and the learning process as had the kindergarten teacher these parents had just visited?

"But what's the point?" Barbara interjects. "How can teachers stay positive when they are given too much to deal with, such as kids with so many problems? That young man who was school-phobic may have had learning or emotional problems that were affecting *his* school attitude." Barbara likely is right. But if he had been treated positively, despite any problems he had, chances are that he would have felt much better about entering the building and starting another year of learning. Student attitudes toward learning develop largely from teacher attitudes about teaching. And students with learning and behavioral problems may require even more positive interactions than students without problems. For children, much more than adults, tend to generalize from a given situation. If adults are in a university class and dislike the professor's teaching style, they still may like the course content and the university itself. Children are different. What they perceive now seems to be typical of everywhere and certainly will last forever. The young man refusing to enter the school building had experienced enough negativism in the rooms inside to generalize to the whole educational process. And he was refusing to be part of it anymore.

Barbara protests, "But I really am a positive person you know, not some Scrooge. I always wanted to be a teacher, and as you've said, while I had a few really negative experiences, most of my teachers were good and made me feel good about myself. My first few years of teaching I was so excited—but I've lost it. Is there any way to rejuvenate an attitude?"

Absolutely. Positive or negative teacher attitudes can stem from a variety of factors, and the best way to effect an attitude change is to isolate the factors having the greatest influence. Sometimes personality or temperament factors are important, where a teacher has more emotional energy and is a markedly happy person. Yet, there is so much more.

POSITIVE TEACHING

Positive teachers usually feel that many of their needs for professional competency and success are being met through their job situation. They are treated with respect by colleagues and administrators and their work is considered important within the school and district. Their positive attitude comes from a sense of acknowledgment by themselves and others of their contributions. They and others feel they are making a difference in young people's lives.

Positive teachers feel that their colleagues in regular education support their work and are receptive to programs for students with learning disabilities. They rarely perceive regular and special education as separate systems trying to divide time with the child. Instead, they feel that educating students with special needs is a combined effort that calls for full cooperation. Positive teachers often view their job as having the primary challenge of smoothly uniting all efforts for child gain. It is difficult not to feel positive when you are working together with colleagues toward tangible goals with students.

Positive teachers feel trained to do their job. Teachers of students with handicapping conditions must feel competent in their awareness of direct teaching methods to use with students. They need to have a facility with a number of instructional techniques, behavioral management systems, and materials. By virtue of their referral for special education services, students will not have learned academics by traditional methods and will need specialized assistance. Special education instructors must have a "bag of tricks" for students who learn differently. Teachers who are comfortable with a variety of instructional methods are less likely to feel threatened by students with unusual learning styles.

Positive teachers have fulfilling personal lives outside the school. When fulfilled by their own family's love and support, it is so much easier for teachers to share these feelings with the people with whom they interact daily. Worried or tired teachers cannot be positive with their students or colleagues and cannot give the concentration necessary to help demanding students. While some teachers insist that they need to take home their lesson plan preparations or papers to score each evening, when they do this, they are depriving themselves and their family of their time. Knowing they have spent enjoyable hours with their spouse or children the evening before is critical to the attitude teachers bring to school the next day.

The critical issue behind this discussion of teachers with positive attitudes is that they come to school satisfied with themselves, their personal lives, and importantly, their jobs, so that they have no need to control students, but are happy to direct them through the learning process. They can concentrate on the "meat" of education because students respond with respect to their efforts. Student attitude is directly related to teacher attitude. Classrooms with positive, Directive Teachers tend to contain positive, cooperative students.

Students pick up all kinds of messages from teachers. Just as teachers informally understand the degree of respect they receive from their building principal, so students understand how much they are respected as individuals. Directive Teachers are truly "resource" teachers and view their role as guiding and supporting students. Consequently, students feel the security and important boundaries of working in a structured environment, yet understand the sense of teacher confidence in their abilities to make choices and to learn independently.

Controlling Teachers are more negative. The message sent to students is that they are not capable of more independent learning, that they must be told what to do with limited choices. This element of control demonstrates a lack of respect for student capabilities and results in a sense of "learned helplessness," where students become dependent on teachers because they feel they cannot be entrusted with their own learning progress.

This feeling is a basic contradiction to a primary goal in education: the creation of independence.

The specific attitude toward learning is very pervasive. Within moments of entering a new classroom the teacher's attitude is apparent, even if observers never speak to the teacher but only watch the students. Children and teenagers model adult behaviors and feelings. And, as discussed earlier, they tend to overgeneralize their own attitudes to the entire learning environment based on individual experiences. When teachers are positive and directive instead of controlling, students "catch" this attitude and become more positive themselves. Within minutes after the beginning of the school day, it is clear to most adults and children whether this is going to be a "good" or "bad" day. Students in the positive environment of a Directive Teacher usually evidence a spirit of cooperation and responsiveness. They tend to have a sense that education is good and that learning can be meaningful and fun. In short, they enjoy school more, often embrace even difficult tasks enthusiastically, and evidence fewer behavioral problems because they respect a teacher who respects them.

On the other hand, in a Controlling Teacher's class the students usually are less motivated. There are often more complaints about tasks and more negative verbal interchanges between teacher and student. Teachers give more orders and students object more about following them. Students tend to be less cooperative because they feel they are not regarded highly by the teacher; subsequently, there are more discipline problems because of a lack of student commitment to the task.

Barbara notes, "My observation is that most people start out their teaching careers with a positive and idealistic attitude and would prefer to be directive instead of controlling. It's not as if you wake up one morning and you've become negative and inflexible overnight. There seems to be a continuum of attitudes, and as the world of problem children and lack of community support reaches our rooms, we move pretty quickly toward the negative end. I do wonder if we can ever get our excitement and enthusiasm back. How do you become a positive, Directive Teacher once you've burned out?"

TAKING CHARGE IN THE CLASSROOM

Whether you enter the classroom as a new teacher, or like Barbara, as a more weathered than seasoned veteran, there are some steps basic to good teaching that you can follow to take charge and maintain the pleasure of teaching. Taking charge requires *knowledge*: about students and their academic functioning levels, their specific learning problems, school and family history, achievement test scores, and behavior. With this knowledge, you can set goals for student performance and then design instructional methods to meet these goals. The following steps should help you begin this process.

Identifying Student Achievement Levels

To design appropriate assignments, teachers must know at what levels their students are functioning. All too often teachers attend a few days of general inservice training sessions before the beginning of school, decorate the bulletin boards, organize existing materials, and feel they are ready to greet their students for the new year. Nothing could be further from the truth. Teachers are never ready to begin the year's instruction until they know what the assessment data reports about students' learning styles and levels.

The first step is to review all previous test data. If assigned to your room, the student should already have an extensive file of diagnostic information completed by the school psychologist or diagnostician stating the student's eligibility for special education. Although I.Q. indicates what to expect in a broad capability level, academic information is more important to the educator, who may want to ask the following questions.

What results demonstrate that the student actually does have a learning disability? Is there a large discrepancy between potential and achievement? Is there a severe disability in one or more academic areas? What appears to be the underlying cause of the learning problem (for example, a disability in receptive language processing, memory, or perception of symbols)?

What academic areas are affected most strongly that will impact on school progress (for example, reading, spelling, arithmetic)? Which performance areas supportive to learning have also been affected (for example, fine or gross motor skills)? Are there "hidden handicaps" such as listening or reading comprehension, association and categorization of new ideas, that may influence performance?

What are the students' strongest learning areas? What are suggested teaching methods and ways of structuring the classroom? Are there behaviors present, such as a short attention span or hyperactivity, which will impact on how much a student will learn? Initially, is there a cooperative family, or will the school have to make the first overtures for supportive interactions?

Working with Appraisal Staff

However, teachers are justifiably frustrated at the diagnostic process. Although the testing for placement into special education likely was done by a trained professional, often the report does not contain useful information for the classroom. Results may have been written in professional, psychological jargon, and even the diagnosis may be difficult to interpret. And since many school psychologists and diagnosticians have never taught children, recommendations at the conclusion of testing often are general and provide no new insights into additional teaching strategies. In many schools, in-depth testing of students does little more than meet state requirements for placement. This awareness often leads to negativism on the part of teachers who feel they are not given enough information to begin teaching a child even after the appraisal is completed.

But educators can take charge in this area as well. First, instead of tolerating this situation, they should communicate with appraisal staff about what they need. They should note that the reports are written in jargon or that they do not contain enough suggestions for specific classroom teaching. Appraisal staff and teachers rarely get together until the final placement meeting, where appraisal staff give a formal report which parents and teachers may not understand, and they then leave quickly to test another student. Yet many people in appraisal have noted that they actually would prefer working more closely with teachers and the families.

Teachers should meet with colleagues doing an appraisal before the child is tested. They should explain the learning and behavioral problems they perceive, invite the school psychologist or diagnostician to informally observe the child in class before beginning testing. The testing situation should replicate the student's classroom setting as closely as possible to achieve the most accurate picture of actual performance.

Educators should be sure that they understand the cause of any disability and ongoing conditions or behaviors as stated in the testing report. For example, there may be discussion of the child having experienced neurological trauma at an early age, resulting in difficulties in receptive language and having direct implication for the student's ability to understand lectures or follow directions; there may have been recurrent ear infections, subsequently causing problems in learning phonics; or the student may be experiencing depression, further lowering school performance. Educators who understand the nature of the student's problem are better equipped to help remediate or compensate.

Regular and special education teachers and appraisal staff should work together to apply the information learned to follow-up classroom teaching techniques and activities. If teachers have questions about the student's ongoing performance after the assessment has been completed, they should work as a team with the appraisal staff person who performed the testing.

But some educators may feel they cannot make these changes in the formal appraisal system because of the size or the policies of their school district. There are many additional sources of information that they can review easily to give them a more complete picture of where their students are functioning and why their skills and behaviors may be problematic.

Moran (1978) details a number of sources of diagnostic information for regular education classroom teachers. These sources range from a thorough review of school records and careful observations of school work products to daily incidental observations. This information can be adapted to meet the needs of teachers of students with learning disabilities.

Reviewing Student Records

Although many teachers initially may feel that records in students' files do not provide enough in-depth information, it is surprising how much can be learned from a careful review. Instead of considering each school year's grades as a single entity, it is helpful to determine any patterns of grades over the previous years. Students with disabilities in some academic areas such as word attack skills or arithmetic computation likely will have demonstrated these problems since first grade. Yet others with problems in reading comprehension, spelling, or written expression often will not begin to have difficulties until third grade when these skills are emphasized. Attentional disabilities such as short attention span and distractibility should have been present from earlier years if they are neurologically based.

It is important to note when a student received average or higher grades in early years but suffered lower grades during a certain school year. It is possible that there may have been an emotional trauma, such as divorce, which influenced performance. If the student's grades did not improve after that time but remained low, emotional responses still may be present. It would be very helpful for the teacher to understand what happened during that period. While this is not always possible, if the child is still at the same school, the teacher can inquire about the situation from the child's teacher during the year when grades declined. It may be possible for the current teacher to work with the school counselor or other personnel to give the child support when there is a continuing emotional problem.

School attendance records also are very important to the understanding of current student functioning levels. Were there numerous absences during the first three years of school when most basic skills are taught? Were most absences during winter months, indicating potential hearing, oral language, and reading problems based on upper respiratory or middle ear infections? Are there numerous records of tardiness in school arrivals, possibly indicating a disorganized family structure? Are there health records attached indicating a problem with hearing or vision, or that the child has asthma and may be medicated heavily at times?

A difficult experience regarding the value of reading health records occurred in a middle school class containing students with a variety of learning problems. The health records were kept in a separate file from other school records and being busy with large daily classes, the teacher did not have the time to read them. One day while showing students a filmstrip and moving the knob quickly, flashing through a number of pictures, the teacher was shocked when one of the students had a grand mal seizure, responding to the brightly flashing images. The other students screamed and were horrified watching this young woman who was their friend and classmate. After helping her through the seizure, the teacher took her to the nurse's office and, upset, asked why she had not been told about the student's history of seizures. The nurse commented that all the information was in the student's record—and indeed it was. Despite subsequent efforts to help the other students understand seizures and how to give their classmate support, afterwards the girl was quietly shunned by the group who at times made fun of her behavior during the seizure. The entire incident could have been avoided if the teacher had read the records and known about her condition in advance or had initiated a process in the school whereby teachers would be notified about serious health conditions.

To understand students' backgrounds and needs, educators also should consider the number and location of schools a student has attended. While there may be many reasons for a family to relocate, such as job changes or military employment, moving usually is disruptive to a child's learning and emotional states. Moving has become such a common phenomenon that some of our inner-city schools report that between one-third and one-half of their students starting the school year will not be there when the year ends. This factor alone is debilitating to teachers who find it disheartening to work hard teaching students who may be moving away at any time. And new students with very difficult learning and emotional problems may appear in classes at any time without prerequisite information necessary to learn the material.

Did this child move frequently? Was it during the early school years, perhaps when basic reading or arithmetic skills may have been disrupted by teachers using completely different approaches? Additionally, frequent moves may have hindered the student's ability or desire to make new friends who might be lost during the next move, causing a sense of distrust and behavior problems.

Moran (1978) notes that many files may include anecdotal records written by the student's former teachers which may contain important information about the child's learning and behavioral history. However, it is necessary to be careful to avoid bias in considering others' comments about students since it may cloud personal responses. For example, as school starts, if a teacher learns from the records that a young man in this year's class can be disruptive by not raising his hand or by talking to others during class, there may be a negative response to him from the beginning, actually encouraging negativism from him because of the teacher's own attitude. Yet, it may have been

the previous year's teacher's lack of class control or the combination of students in that class that triggered the disruptions.
It would be far better to provide a structured environment and
to give him a chance in a new situation. On the other hand, a
teacher may have written that he tends to have problems concentrating on subject matter or in making friends. These comments might give some hints as to where to locate his desk in
the room or to be sure to include him in social interactions.

But responses to students should never come from comments made by others in the Faculty Lounge. If a teacher would
like to regain a positive attitude, it might be best to avoid staff
who complain about students (and everything else) in favor of
a few trusted colleagues whose opinions are well-considered.

The same concern about bias might be part of the way that
a teacher reviews I.Q. scores in student records. There has been
enough controversy to keep some districts from publishing I.Q.
scores because of questions about their validity with certain groups
of students. While this concern has focused primarily on performance by students from lower socioeconomic groups or from
different ethnic backgrounds, there should be greater concern
about the validity of I.Q. instruments for students with learning
disabilities. As indicated in Figure 1-4, results from an individually
administered test may indicate strengths and weaknesses in specific
cognitive processes such as sequencing or symbol encoding,
causing a diminished score in the overall I.Q. because of lower
scores in specific areas. Ironically, while I.Q. subtests can be quite
accurate in isolating the actual disability area, their combination
into Verbal, Performance, and clearly, Full-Scale scores may not
give a true indicator of the student's skills because of the strength
of a single disability area on the combined score. In other words,
students with learning disabilities often obtain lower combined
scores on these tests than might be indicated by their actual
intelligence (Waldron & Saphire, 1990).

Therefore, a teacher might look to individual I.Q. subtest
results as indicators of a student's stronger and weaker learning
areas, but should not necessarily believe that the total I.Q. score
is a valid mark of the student's potential. Too often, noting an
I.Q. of 90 or 100 encourages teachers to put limits on how
much they feel a student actually can learn.

What about other standardized test scores? While they may
provide a standard of student performance based on norms, they

often provide too little information for the classroom teacher. As Moran (1978) notes:

> The major limitation of published individual tests of achievement is not the construction of such tests or the skill of the teacher in administering them, but rather their variance from the tasks the student is asked to perform each day in a specific classroom. (p. 30)

It may be of interest to know that a student is in the ninth percentile nationally in word attack skills, but unless there is specific information about what has and has not been learned, this information does not help teachers.

However, standardized tests can be useful if the results include the actual student booklets so that teachers can tell which skills students do and do not have. Teachers should ask to have student record booklets returned to them for review as a basis of content for incorporation into their curriculum. For example, knowing that students are performing below expectancy in phonics generally does not help the teacher plan a specific lesson; knowing that students are having difficulty with certain consonant blends and digraphs does help them plan. The specific problem areas can be found by reviewing the individual test items and then grouping students for instruction based on areas of need. If results are to be useful, standardized tests should be given early in the fall and results returned to teachers; if the district does not wish to change its spring test administration period, then the student record booklets should be given to the next year's teacher.

Examining Work Products and Observing Informal Behavior

Often too much credence appears to be given to standardized instruments and not enough credence to teachers' informal observations. Although it may be true in some instances that teachers newer to the profession are more innovative and excited about teaching, those who have taught longer often have a better norm perspective by understanding what should be typical behavior of, for example, a third grader. They are able to look at a student's daily work or behavior and quickly and informally diagnose where the problems may be.

Teachers can use clues to tell why and where the student is lagging behind. Does the student have problems following

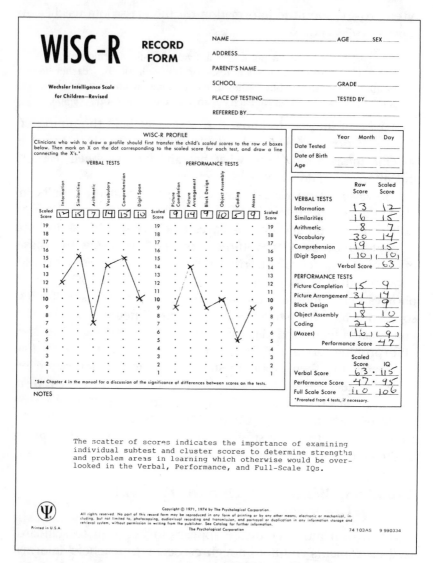

Figure 1-4. WISC-R profile of a student with learning disabilities. Wechsler Intelligence Scale for Children-Revised. Copyright© 1974 by The Psychological Corporation. Reproduced by permission. All rights reserved.

oral directions and/or written ones? Can the student finish work as quickly as others in the class or is there a problem with rate? Is the student organized, or are papers frequently lost or assignments forgotten? Can the student finish as much work as others in a given time or is there a constant time pressure with rare completion of assignments?

Observations can be particularly valuable in academic areas. The teacher should note which students have word attack problems or a low "sight word" vocabulary in their oral reading. With older students, which ones tend to misunderstand passages and to forget facts? Are errors in arithmetic a result of basic computational mistakes, and if so, in which operations? Do spelling errors form a pattern such as letter missequencing, or does the student only misspell nonphonetic words? Teachers should look for fine motor skill problems including how the student holds the pencil and forms letters on the page. How is material organized on the page? Does the student have problems writing on the line or keeping numbers and letters the same size? In arithmetic problems, are numbers aligned well in columns or is it difficult for the student to discern which numbers are being added or subtracted because of the way they are spaced on the page?

Informal observations also can indicate which of the errors are caused by the actual learning disability and which are the result of carelessness or hurry to finish. While everyone makes careless errors at times, students with learning disabilities particularly are prone to problems based on disorganization and impulsivity. Student work early in the day may differ dramatically from afternoon performance or assignments completed after physical education or recess, where both quality and quantity are lessened.

Once assessment data are examined, the teacher should set goals for student performance. Too often goal-setting is treated as if it is unrelated to assessment. It is important to remember that test results by themselves mean nothing, but it is what is done with them that is significant. Once teachers know where students' strengths and weaknesses lie, teaching becomes less threatening and a sense of direction is developed. Years ago, when educational theorists tended to support the Behaviorism of Skinner and Mager, each student problem area was examined carefully and an objective was established, measured by observable behaviors that the student would demonstrate to indicate achievement. Evaluation criteria were based on expectation of the student performing the behavior at a specified level of accuracy and frequency. The Behaviorist emphasis taught educators to specify what was being measured and to gauge criteria of success based on observable behaviors rather than on more general and difficult-to-measure goals such as "knowledge" and "understanding." It also provided a degree of comfort to know long-term goals for each child.

Currently, teachers have worked to humanize this approach. As a teacher of students with learning disabilities recently shared, "Of course I want my students to form their letters more accurately when they write—that's an important goal so that others can read their work. But it's more important that I instill in them a desire to write, a love of writing. While it's so much more difficult to measure, I can tell when they're finally hooked just by their excitement and pleasure. I would go crazy trying to measure this enjoyment exactly, but I can certainly tell when it's there."

While the administrative system has sought to formalize the process of goal setting by having teachers complete extensive paperwork, effective educators usually know where they are going with student instruction and at what performance levels they want their students to be at the completion of instruction. Since formal assessment data must be available as part of placement criteria for all students with learning differences, a basis is provided for knowing current performance levels. Instead of calling on appraisal staff for additional assessment after placement, teachers and supportive staff should conduct continuous evaluation of student performance after the initiation of remedial work. Educators should turn to appraisal staff if puzzled about lack of student progress or if needing additional help with teaching strategies to better reach students.

As will be discussed in Chapter 3, grouping is an important basis for classroom instruction. Once students have been placed in small groups with students of similar instructional needs, teaching goals can be formulated for the group instead of for individual students. For example, the goal for one group might be to improve reading comprehension of main ideas in paragraphs, while the goal for another group could be to work on spelling patterns in words, and the goal for a third group could be to properly divide fractions in math. Although most teachers believe they cannot be working on this many subject areas at any one time, it is more efficient than trying to meet goals for students by teaching them as one large group when their needs are dramatically different. And importantly, educators regain enthusiasm and a positive attitude by knowing they actually are teaching students what they need to know.

Building Positive Expectations

The teacher should work together with other faculty and the principal to create an optimistic mood about students with special needs. Children behave at the level of expectations: If adults in the school convey the message that students are not capable of learning more academics or improved behaviors, the students themselves will feel they cannot change. But if the environment states loudly that "In this building, all students, regardless of class placement, are competent," students mirror what adults expect.

A number of years ago, a new teacher faced a very difficult assignment: a self-contained classroom for students with severe learning disabilities, mental retardation, or emotional disturbance, ages 10 to 15 years, located in a public elementary school with only one other special education unit for less-problemed, younger children. The students in the class were feared by most teachers and students, but especially by the principal, who had loudly protested the district's decision to place this unit in her building. In fairness, the concern had some justification, since the classroom was the "last stop" for these children, many of whom would be sent to a state institution if they could not learn appropriate behaviors and some academics. A few of the students had a history of violent behavior, but the rest largely were children of poverty, abuse, and neglect, with little stimulation in their homes. Their neighborhood, "the Courts," was a common scene of violence and substance abuse, with children reporting that they often stepped over the bodies of drunks as they walked to school in the morning.

The main problem appeared to be that the children had no normalcy in their lives, little healthy adult or peer behaviors from which to model. It seemed that if the school could provide examples of positive, directive, structured behaviors with predictable outcomes on top of stimulation and communication, these children really could be helped. But ironically, the school, the very place to provide these models, isolated these students from others out of fear. And the leader of the school, the principal, not only supported this isolation, but sought to broaden it.

The principal viewed a successful classroom as orderly, traditional and, above all, quiet. At weekly faculty meetings, she praised certain teachers and their rooms, usually commenting with sarcasm about the behavior of students in the "retarded class." With nothing to lose, the new teacher began a simple behavior modification program in her classroom, rewarding students with a cookie each time an adult entered the room and they became quiet, sitting in the seats where they were completing small-group or individual assignments. Amusingly, the principal often would open the classroom door at least several times a week to observe student behavior. After the system was in place, and student behavior was quiet and orderly, she observed daily, sometimes even stopping in a few times in one day. Students would comment to each other, "She's here!" and become silent. After she left, all cooperative students were rewarded. Hungry ones often were heard to ask, "Where is she?" Within a few weeks, the principal's attitude began to change, and she mentioned at a faculty meeting that some of the teachers might want to look at the behavior of these students, commenting "If even the retarded class can behave, what's the problem with some of the others?" After the first month of acknowledged improved behavior, the teacher moved forward with her campaign.

She asked the principal if, on a trial basis, her students could be allowed to eat in the lunchroom with the students in nonspecial classes, something that had never been tried before. While extremely reluctant, the principal agreed, as long as the students sat in a separate section ("so no one would be hurt") and maintained their appropriate behavior. The class practiced for days how they would behave around the other students, later practiced how they would behave in school assembly programs from which they had been excluded, and next, during recess on the playground with other students. The progress was not always smooth, and occasionally students had to be removed from the setting because of misbehavior, facing very strong consequences from the teacher.

But the message had become clear, to the principal and other teachers, but most importantly, to the students themselves. They could do it. They could behave acceptably after all.

The more often they were integrated successfully, the stronger the normalization message became. When the art, music, and physical education teachers were asked if a few of the students, carefully selected, might participate in their regular classes, they agreed, although with hesitation. The teacher personally monitored student progress, weekly talking with mainstream teachers and students placed in their classes, making continued participation in the regular education program the reward for a student's efforts at appropriate behaviors.

The project was successful because the educators in the school all had an attitude change caused by working together toward a common goal. Too often teachers of students with special needs complain about the lack of understanding and respect they and their students receive, based on the principal's and other teachers' reluctance to accept them wholeheartedly into the mainstream of school activities. It is clear that to initiate change and create a positive attitude toward the students, special educators must take the lead.

DIRECTING THE INSTRUCTIONAL VARIABLES

But Barbara, as always, brings us back to reality. "These are lovely thoughts about developing a positive attitude, and I certainly can't disagree, but I've still got kids in my classroom every day who won't even sit in their seats. My attitude will improve greatly when they can pay attention for more than 5 minutes. Suggestions, please."

Barsch (1965), a pioneer in learning disabilities, suggested a number of factors that the teacher can direct to provide an environment in which students optimally can learn despite a number of Attention Deficit Disorder problems. These factors, discussed in the following paragraphs, allow teachers to take charge of student performance by creating a flexible setting in which a variety of individual student behavioral needs are met.

Space

Many students whose learning disabilities are neurologically based have an adverse response to large, open work areas. They seem to become overly stimulated and unable to attend. At times, students who are severely impaired will attempt to steady themselves in the more open building areas, apparently experiencing a sense of disequilibrium. Yet, when these same students work in study carrels they can complete their work effectively and with drastically improved attention. Students even appear to complete their work better when at small desks than at larger tables.

Although students cannot sit at study carrels all day, teachers might direct them to limited space areas for deskwork requiring optimal concentration in academic areas. Additionally, natural room partitions can be used to modify space. For example, a student's desk might be placed next to a filing cabinet or bookcase or partitions used for a learning center. In this way, students can participate in large-group activities in a spatially limited environment in which they may feel more secure.

Because some students become more hyperactive and distractible when their seatwork is performed in the main classroom area, teachers can create their own study carrels by bringing in television cartons and putting each on top of a student's desk by the wall in a quiet area. The teacher and students remove one side of the box, allowing the remaining three sides to provide an enclosed area that inhibits visual distractions. Calling them "offices," a status title, the teacher can explain to students that everyone has certain tasks such as reading, spelling, and math which require increased concentration and could be better performed in a quiet area. Students should be directed to sign up for an office when they are involved in one of these tasks. Students most affected by distractibility should be encouraged to sign up more frequently. The most common problem educators face with these carrels is having to create more to meet student demand.

Students cannot stay cloistered forever, even when space reduction has become an effective means of increasing their attention to task. The amount of space within which students are required to work must be increased gradually so they will be able to perform well in a work environment some day. This expansion beyond limited space can begin by helping them take control of their own personal space needs. At first, educators can encourage students to use carrels or to sit in a limited space environment based on personal observations of when students are most distracted or require the most concentration. As students begin to succeed, they can move gradually to a larger space area, such as a learning center or table in a corner of the room. Eventually, they should be able to relocate to the center of the classroom. It is important to realize that this progress may take months or even years, making it critical that teachers work together as a team to provide consistency. The final goal is that through such practice, students will begin to internalize their controls to participate in an unmodified environment.

Time

Teachers in regular and special education commonly complain that students with learning disabilities rarely finish their work. Often the problem does not appear to lie in a lack of understanding of the task or an unwillingness to perform, but in a short attention span. Again, the teacher can direct the environment to allow for time flexibility. When students are hyperactive or inattentive after a short period, they can be given breaks, for example, to get a drink of water or bring the work already completed to the teacher. Although teachers often tend to discontinue a task when a student becomes fidgety, this action may not be necessary. Many times, even after a break of one or two minutes, students are able to return to a task feeling refreshed.

On the other hand, at times students do need to have assignments shortened. Educators need to remember that there is nothing sacred about a textbook, and often the amount of material contained on a page or in a unit is based more on printing costs than on any other factor. Partial-page or even one-line assignments may be appropriate for some students. Workbooks also can pose problems because the amount of space allotted may not be enough for students with difficulties in visual-spatial or visual-motor skills, who may formulate letters of different sizes and organize them poorly on the page (see Figure 1-5). It often is best to cut out sections of workbook pages for students or to allow them the space they need on separate sheets of paper.

Preconceptions about how long it *should* take to complete an assignment will have to change, especially since the final goal is quality. Often, students with learning disabilities cannot learn to spell 10 or 20 spelling words for Friday's test, but they can learn to spell 5 or 6 in one week. Or they may not be able to

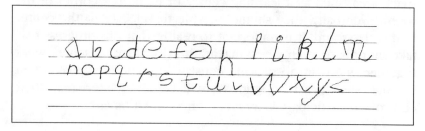

Figure 1-5. Writing of a student with visual-spatial and visual-motor problems.

complete the math test in 20 minutes, but they would be able to complete it in 30 minutes. Success is more important than speed.

Timing of activities also is important. Regardless of attention span, anyone gets tired and bored if expected to sit quietly for a long time doing seatwork. Teachers should vary quiet and lively activities, thereby demanding less continuous concentration and allowing students to return renewed after a break which may actually have been work in another area, such as studying fractions through reading a cookbook or learning concepts through a song.

Number of Factors

Students with learning disabilities often are overloaded. As Smith (1981) notes, they tend to be confused and suffer cognitive disorganization when attempting to integrate new ideas. Adding the Attention Deficit Hyperactivity Disorder characteristics of distractibility to visual, auditory, and/or tactile stimuli, they appear to be bombarded by constant bits of environmental information that becomes overwhelmingly difficult to process.

Because these factors may be out of student control, teachers must modify the environment to limit the numbers of factors to which students are exposed at any one time. Students may perform better when only the paperwork they are completing is on their desk, even when they have a standard style pen or pencil instead of a more stimulating one with varied colors or adjustments to distract them.

Frequent schedule changes should be avoided since students rely on consistency as a basis for integrating organization. Many students with special needs respond poorly to changing classes and teachers, especially when such changes necessitate moving around the building and dealing with different behavioral and teaching methods. Often students indeed are creatures of habit and do not respond well to factors of change. Although they cannot adhere rigidly to artificial structures in school and later be able to adapt to the adult world, they can be moved gradually through changes, introducing one change at a time.

Although some early experts in learning disabilities urged that the environment essentially be sterile in decor, this philosophy has not been embraced by most current teachers, who tend to prefer warmth and color as a basis for a supportive atmosphere. However, in most effective classrooms there still exist areas that are less decorated and distracting as an acknowledgment that some students will not respond well to an overly stimulating environment.

Difficulty

Students with poor word attack skills cannot read advanced texts any more than students who cannot perform fractions can be successful in geometry. No one does well at tasks that are too difficult. While specific ways of dealing with academic diversity within the classroom will be discussed in the next chapter, it is important for teachers to adhere to the principle that students should *never* be given work above their current ability level. When students know they cannot be successful in a task, they refuse to try, with the result often being a negative attitude and behaviors that are disruptive to others. Adolescents most often respond by not completing in-class assignments or homework so that they can boast to friends that they "didn't feel like doing it," instead of admitting publically that they could not do it. No one likes to feel stupid.

While students intellectually may be at a level of understanding concepts, they may not have the prerequisite skills to succeed in applying new ideas. Middle and high school teachers often complain that although they want to teach content subjects, they rarely can, because many students come to them unprepared to learn new information because of low basic skills. Unfortunately, too often these teachers refuse to review prerequisites because it is "not their job." So the student sits in their classrooms unprepared to learn the information, wasting everyone's time and often causing behavioral problems stemming from a sense of personal frustration.

Students with learning disabilities are frequently in this situation, even in special education classrooms where they should be receiving remediation. As discussed earlier, it is important for teachers to review previous assessment data and to rely heavily on their ongoing personal observations of student work products as a basis for teaching missing skills and giving students assignments at their level and at which they can be successful. Once this process begins, teachers will be amazed at the lessening of behavioral problems and the improvement of student motivation to complete their assignments.

Language

The fact that "Learning Disabilities" as a diagnostic classification originally was often called "Language-Learning Disabilities" underscores the frequency of language disruption as a basis for learning problems. Educators may need to change the way they use language in the classroom to improve student learning. For example, many students do not follow directions because they cannot understand them or because they are distracted by auditory or visual stimuli in the classroom.

Fortunately, most teachers are kind and caring. Subsequently, when speaking to students they use words like "Please," "Thank you," and usually expand verbally on subject matter so that students will fully understand material. While these are positive practices, they often use language beyond the receptive capabilities of many students with language disabilities. Teachers need to become more "telegraphic" in speech patterns, a trait with which they often do not feel comfortable. For many students, less talk during teaching is far better than expanded explanations where words become a jumble and difficult to understand.

Shorter sentences with fewer adverbs and clauses tend to be more effective. Teachers should avoid a passive structure in speaking (for example, students better understand "He threw the ball" than "The ball was thrown by him"). Sentences using negative constructions may be equally difficult ("It is not unusual"). Words with multiple meanings, colloquialisms, or abstract terms that cannot be interpreted literally should not be used, because students may have difficulty with interpretation.

When speaking, teachers should be brief, direct, and "to-the-point." Instead of saying, "Class, please sit down now so that I can check your work and we can start to get ready for lunch," the teacher might say, "Class, go to your seats now." When students are seated, the teacher can add, "Put your papers on your desk." Whether talking to individuals or groups, teachers will find that using gestures will provide a strong support for understanding.

When needing the attention of the entire class, teachers should have a preset signal, such as flashing the lights several times or ringing a bell, which alerts students to the need to pay attention. No instructions should be given until everyone is seated and quiet. To be assured that individual students have understood directions, teachers might quietly go to these students' desks after the class has begun their work and have them repeat the instructions.

While giving directions, teachers should be sure that students are looking directly at them. If a student is so distracted that maintaining eye contact is impossible, teachers might gently put their thumb under the student's chin to keep the head from turning away. Even this may not work with children who are severely neurologically impaired, as their eyes may keep looking away as you hold their chin. By gently putting your hands on the side of the student's head thereby holding the head steady and blocking out other visual input, you will be able to obtain full attention and have them accurately repeat and carry out instructions. You can fade this technique, going next to the holding of the chin, then only to calling students' names for attention. Although the process may take months, students will be able to internalize controls and eventually to better attend.

Since many children have problems recalling and sequencing information heard, teachers should limit directions and verbalizations to student recall levels. For example, if John can remember only one direction at a time, at first he should be given only one ("John, put your books away"). To expand his recall, the teacher gradually should add a second related, easy-to-follow direction ("John, put your books away and sit down"), followed eventually by a less-related second command ("John, put your books away and go to the Math Center"). After the student begins to show facility for following two commands, the teacher can add a third, expecting that at first the student may missequence directions.

As part of keeping our classrooms positive and students motivated, teachers should explain (briefly) that their goal is to have students become better listeners. Students should be praised for attending and following directions instead of criticized for "not listening."

SUMMARY

In this chapter, discussion included how the academic needs of students with learning disabilities differ from those of other students. Learning disabilities are noted to exist in a wide variety of areas with teachers needing to consider specific learning strengths and problems of the student and not to rely on a less definitive category title which may not describe actual learning behaviors.

Barbara, a teacher with problems faced by most educators today, has noted the incredible spectrum of behaviors and problems students are bringing to today's classrooms and has asked for suggestions in preventing burnout by teachers who clearly are feeling overwhelmed. In response, a redesign of the classroom was suggested, putting teachers back in charge of learning, yet doing so in the midst of a positive environment where they can become enthusiastic and feel successful. Bases for positive teaching included teachers feeling that their needs for professional competency and success are being met through their job situation, that they are supported by colleagues in regular education, that they are trained to do their jobs well, and that their own personal lives are fulfilling.

Some prerequisites were suggested to allow teachers to "take charge" in their classrooms, including: a review of all previous assessment data; ongoing interactions with appraisal staff; a careful review of school history from patterns of grades over the years to health and attendance records; understanding the meaning of intelligence tests and standardized achievement measures; and careful observation of daily work products and behavior.

Goal-setting also was included as an important basis for indicating where efforts should be directed, and emphasis was placed on the need to work together with colleagues to achieve these goals.

Because of the high incidence of behavioral concerns in classes for students with learning disabilities, suggestions were made to redirect instructional variables, including reducing work space; creating flexibility in the amount time students are allowed to co-plete their work; limiting the number of stimuli distracting students; adjusting assignment difficulty to the student's achievement level; and simplifying teacher verbal language to avoid overloading students.

Chapter 2 includes discussion of specific classroom organizational strategies, focusing on learner needs within learning diversity.

Chapter 2

ORGANIZING THE CLASSROOM FOR SUCCESS

It is impossible to describe the "typical" classroom for students with learning disabilities today, largely because of the shifting philosophies regarding optimal instruction. Barbara has been teaching in the more traditional resource room setting favored in her district, where she works with most students for 50 minutes a day. She is viewed as the expert in helping children with exceptional needs and, similar to many other special education teachers, she has developed an "unwritten contract" (Gallagher, 1991) with colleagues in regular education: they will send their problem learners to her daily and she will perform her magic to cure them. As part of this contract, regular class teachers do not have to learn additional instructional and behavioral management methods and, for her part, Barbara is permitted to work with fewer students, supported by additional materials, and acknowledged by others as being "patient" and "caring."

The resource room allows students to participate with their peers in the mainstream classroom for most of the day, while still providing an environment for basic skills remediation. Its success depends on a number of variables: knowledge of an array of techniques by the specialist, a collaborative relationship between special and regular education teachers to assure reinforcement of skills development across the curriculum, scheduling, supportive materials and equipment, and a positive interaction with parents. But within the resource classroom, the teacher must be able to concentrate on skills development because student time in the room is so limited.

It is clear that individual programming is needed to solve individual student problems. However, the traditional model of combining students with dissimilar (or even similar) disabilities for a brief period of time daily with a specialized teacher has not worked in most school districts. Despite even a specific diagnosis of similar learning problems, when students are placed together, too often the teacher finds that they are at dramatically differing severity levels of the problem, with learning and/or behavioral styles that are incompatible for the students to be able to work together.

As a result, instructional models for serving students with learning disabilities are changing. As so many school districts currently are finding, the resource classroom with a teacher isolated from colleagues and expected to "cure" difficult educational and social problems is not only unrealistic, but is failing. Family problems combined with a learning disability are too much for any one teacher to handle alone. More innovative instructional arrangements, such as "Content Mastery," are becoming popular alternatives for the traditional resource classroom.

CONTENT MASTERY

Content Mastery is an attempt to get away from some of the more problematic areas of the traditional model, such as scheduling and lack of knowledge of remedial strategies by the regular classroom teacher. Although individual schools differ in their implementation, most often students remain in their regular classroom during the presentation of information by the classroom teacher. If they have not understood the information thoroughly, and most frequently, when they need help with reinforcement activities, they go to the Content Mastery teacher, who works with them individually or in a small group to understand and to complete the assignment. Many teachers in regular and special education prefer this model because it allows students to remain in the mainstream classroom and to access help when needed. Therefore, students do not miss valuable class time and information, but are supported in problem areas such as reading the text or completing written work. Since students usually can choose whether to go to the Content Mastery teacher, they are more motivated to work when they do attend.

One of the finest Content Mastery programs is in Carrollton-Farmers Independent School District, near Fort Worth, Texas, and it serves as a model for statewide and national implementation. Its success appears to have been a result of strong cooperation between the regular and special education programs in the district. Teachers in regular education have viewed Content Mastery as a means of supporting their efforts to be successful with a variety of students in their classrooms.

In the district's junior high Content Mastery classrooms, regular education teachers come by to visit the specialist, sharing students' progress. They often stop in to record their exam schedule on a calendar board so that that the Content Mastery teacher can work with several students in advance of the exams, helping them prepare in an orderly fashion. This practice allows the specialist to schedule time to give the test in an alternative manner when necessary. Other mainstream teachers request advice on computer software or additional supportive materials. In this setting, the Content Mastery teacher is a resource both for students and teachers.

Unfortunately, not all Content Mastery programs run as smoothly. Many teachers complain that they feel like tutors. One teacher who is particularly organized and dynamic noted that she misses "teaching." "Every week I plan ahead with the teachers in the school so I know what they will be covering with the students in special education. I have copies of the books and review them in advance so that when a student appears for reinforcement I can help. But I rarely get to teach students the skills they are lacking unless they coincide closely with needs in the assignment. The main emphasis tends to be on finishing homework or studying for an exam, not on skills remediation and compensation. The students do get through their assignments and tests, but there may be little basic skills improvement and I wonder if they will need to be tutored all their academic lives."

For this reason, many schools that had previously embraced Content Mastery as the most exciting of the new directions are altering some pieces of the basic framework. As part of a prereferral process, children now are being screened more carefully for learning problems as they enter school, are placed in a high-risk category, and assigned to academic readiness classes, most commonly in reading and language. These children are not in special education; quite the opposite, they are participating in these classes as an attempt to deal with the learning problem now and to prevent the need for a special education placement later.

Teachers in these early academic programs, such as "Reading Recovery," note that many children make learning strides, especially with one-on-one instruction, but that the classes are too brief, usually meeting for no more than 30 minutes daily. A major problem appears to be that since there are too many of these students, only the ones with the poorest skills can be included. Therefore, there is often a high percentage of students in first and second grade with mild to moderate skill deficiencies who could benefit much more quickly than some of the students in the program, but because of limited resources cannot be included. In most districts, these students remain in regular education classes for a year or two, and when they begin to experience academic problems, they are placed in the Content Mastery program. They are "falling through the cracks" of the system: if intensive work were provided early, they might never experience academic difficulties or need additional support in the future.

DEVELOPING EFFECTIVE PRACTICES

To deal with these concerns, many resource teachers are changing the way they provide model services. Some are keeping resource classes going for students with severe disabilities, while consulting with the mainstream teacher on individual students, or providing direct services within the mainstream classroom to students with learning disabilities.

As educators seek to be innovative and to select the best system for any individual school, *they must start with the child, not the program,* and must examine the individual goal-setting discussed in Chapter 1. Does the child require services more intense than can be met by 30 minutes a day? Are the learning needs so unique and demanding that they are beyond the training of the regular classroom teacher? Are teachers flexible and willing to individualize instruction for differentiated learning, both in the special and regular education units?

There does not appear to be any one system that is optimal for reaching all students with learning disabilities. But there are effective organizational strategies and teaching methods that can affect most students, regardless of degree of regular or special education placement. The "Effective Schools" research (Berliner, 1984; Brophy & Good, 1986; Hunter, 1984; Rosenshine & Stevens, 1986), attempting to identify those teaching practices that resulted in the highest achievement by students, included the following:

1. A focus on academic skill areas under teacher direction, supported by sequenced, structured materials
2. Student understanding of the focus of goals
3. Sufficient time for instruction and follow-up reinforcement
4. Broad content coverage
5. Ongoing evaluation of student work
6. Teacher questions with emphasis on correctness of student responses, and
7. Immediate feedback to students on their academic achievement.

While these elements describe effective teaching of students in regular education, Bickel and Bickel (1986) and Morsink, Soar, Soar, and Thomas (1986) discuss their suitability for students with learning disabilities, emphasizing the need of the teacher to additionally provide structure, to develop a positive emotional climate, and to focus on student-initiated activities as a means of motivation.

The following organizational methods are applicable within a variety of classrooms containing students with learning disabilities: the early referral unit for high-risk children entering school; the traditional resource classroom; the modified Content Mastery class where remediation and compensation are emphasized along with supportive information for classroom instruction; the self-contained unit where students receive highly intense instruction; and the regular education classroom where the teacher may feel overwhelmed by the need to provide education for so many diverse students. While these settings appear very different, they are similar in their need to provide for a variety of learning and behavioral responses.

Teacher-Centered Versus Student-Centered Classrooms

Mrs. Dixon's resource classroom follows a traditional model. Her desk is at the front of the room with students' desks facing her, and she spends most of her instructional time explaining new material to the entire class. Since most of her students have problems in word attack skills, spelling, and arithmetic computation, she teaches these areas based on what the majority of students need to know. Her instruction is usually to the total class, followed by their completion of worksheets at their desk. While Mrs. Dixon notes that some of the children already may know the information, she says that "the reinforcement is good for them." For the students whose achievement level is lower than the content being presented, she says, "Even if they're not ready for it yet, being exposed to this information can't hurt."

Mrs. Dixon does not believe in much small group work or individual work since "Students tend to talk more and work less." She gives written exams at the end of her teaching unit and then begins the next level of instruction. Any student who performs poorly "can come in and ask questions during my free period." She is not surprised that students rarely come in for remedial help since she says that students tend to lack motivation these days.

In addition, Mrs. Dixon has two Content Mastery classes where students come to her room when they need support for information they do not understand in their mainstream room. During these sessions students bring their books and assignments, sit in study carrels in different areas of the room, begin their written work, and ask her questions if they have a problem. She checks on their progress and reads them paragraphs from their book or corrects their arithmetic or grammar and goes on to the next student. Sometimes she reads them questions from a test if requested by the mainstream teacher, but she prefers to have them try to read the questions themselves.

Students in Mrs. Dixon's classes receive checks on a chart for completing their daily work without talking or leaving their seats. By Friday any students with five checks receives some "free time" where they are allowed to listen to music or to visit with a friend. However, she notes that very few of her students earn this reward since they tend to break class rules daily, especially by talking with other students when they are supposed to be working. Recently, since fewer students have been completing their work, she has begun "tightening up" on students by being more strict on her "no talking" rules.

Mrs. Garza teaches by a different philosophy. Her desk is at the side of the classroom and it goes almost unnoticed since she rarely is seated there. Instead she walks about the classroom, responding to raised hands or going directly to a student who appears to have trouble completing the assignment. At times she gives directions to the entire class when there is a large group activity, but this is unusual. Most often, students enter the room, go to the chart with their name on it, note their assignment, and begin. She checks with them briefly to assure that they have understood the directions.

In contrast to Mrs. Dixon's room, there is a moderate level of noise in this room. Kevin and Michael are reading a chapter of a new book into a tape recorder; Jane is at the computer practicing multiplication tables; Juan is reading the financial pages, measuring how much "his" stocks have changed from yesterday as a means of reinforcing fractions. Students' desks are in pairs or in a study carrel for students who do need to work alone for concentration. And the learning centers again are in full use.

Students receive a check mark and three pieces of popcorn for each 20 minutes of cooperative behavior. Depending on how many check marks they have by the end of the week they get to choose which educational game they will play on Friday. (Mrs. Garza does not believe in rewarding the children with time to talk or other noneducational activities, noting that learning can be fun and is its own reward.) In her room there is the positive attitude mentioned earlier. The students are happy and usually cooperative.

Teachers can be directive but still have a student-centered classroom, where the needs of the learner are the most important variable in planning activities. When students feel that they are at the core of the learning process and that the achievement of their academic goals is the top priority, they have a positive attitude and reinforce the teacher's instruction through friendly cooperation even when tasks are difficult. Mrs. Dixon sets the goals at a middle level of student performance and frequently misses the needs of children who are above or below that achievement level. Because students' appraised needs are often in a variety of subject areas—from word attack skills to verbal expressive language to handwriting—there is little hope that a lesson in reading comprehension or spelling is even part of everyone's individualized educational plan. In other words, she is "missing the boat" with many students by not teaching the content that they need.

Additionally, she is ignoring their optimal learning styles. Mrs. Dixon is clearly an auditory learner herself, demonstrated by her tendency to try to explain most information, by lecturing instead of using visual aids or demonstrating her meaning. This tendency for teachers to instruct as they have best learned is common. Educators cannot ignore the fact that students may learn differently and when not instructed through their appropriate learning modalities, they often may learn nothing except frustration. Students respond by boredom, by lack of effort since they realize they will have difficulty understanding, and as they become more distracted, they demonstrate behavior problems.

In Mrs. Garza's room, students cooperate. She does not insist on large-group activity where all students cover the same material. Student goals are evidenced by wall charts stating instructional objectives ("Keith will improve his cursive handwriting") with daily activities listed under them. When Keith goes to the chart each day the goal is reinforced, and he begins activities to support learning in the specified area. When there are other students with similar needs, they are grouped together; if not, he works independently. Mrs. Garza also understands that students with learning disabilities may have even more unique learning styles than other students, and she tries to provide a variety of activities in the classroom. She has visual aids, learning centers that allow for experiences, auditory supports, and where possible multisensory activities. Not only are students studying the content they need, they are learning it through their strongest modality, aiding comprehension and retention.

Barbara interrupts: "Mrs. Garza's room sounds wonderful, but none of us has the time to prepare all those lessons or to set up all those groups. Since we've just discussed the need to teach to students' academic level and attention span, within a modified environment, I feel like I need a telephone booth to change into my Superwoman outfit. I can't afford the time to do all this."

You can't afford not to. Once teachers have a system developed for organizing the classroom, grouping students, and presenting information in a variety of ways, they find it difficult to go back to traditional large-group instruction. (The main reason for this is that students would lose their motivation and their excitement about learning, changing from a positive to a negative classroom attitude.) But teachers cannot make all these changes at once or they would become overwhelmed. One step at a time, Barbara, and the task becomes manageable.

STEP 1: DISCOVERING STUDENT INTERESTS

Many teachers watch students with learning disabilities grumble through their work, struggling to keep up with students in regular classrooms, and it appears natural that their learning has to be negative. While gifted students are expected to become excited about concepts and outcomes, without realizing it, too often the fallacy has been accepted that students with learning differences will learn better if they have more rote practice. In actuality, *students with learning differences learn better if they are interested in what they are doing.* They are no different from anyone else. The most direct way to find out what they are interested in is simply to ask them.

The following "Student Interest Survey" (see Figure 2-1) is directed toward students with learning differences, although many teachers have noted that it can be used with any type of learner. Since students may be participating in a variety of classrooms, questions are included which would help the resource, Content Mastery, and regular education teachers understand not only student preferences for the topics and types of information studied, but also for student learning style and test-taking needs. The survey need only be completed once by the student, and its results can be shared with all involved teachers.

The survey should be administered at the beginning of the school year. While it actually would be preferable for the regular classroom teacher to have students complete it, the teacher of students who are learning disabled usually finds it easier, having fewer students at any one time. Although many students can read the survey themselves, it is far better if the teacher reads it aloud to the students one section at a time so that they will more completely consider each category and will not respond impulsively. In this manner, the teacher also can be assured that students understand the questions. There is a space at the end of each section for students to complete if they have interests or learning needs that have not been included.

The first section of the survey has students identify topics they most enjoy in reading and writing activities. While teachers cannot change textbooks easily, these student preferences can form the basis for additional readings and reports. Since many students with learning disabilities dread written assignments because of skills deficiencies, it is important that they are motivated to do the written reports through motivational topics. Most students cannot handle the lack of structure in a "choose-your-own-topic" assignment, but work best after teachers discover what their interests are and then suggest topics that they have indicated they enjoy.

The second section on the survey asks students the type of literature they prefer. Students who previously have refused to read because of a history of failure show excitement at being allowed to read a magazine about a hobby such as skateboarding. Students with a short attention span often enjoy reading comics or more concrete poetry. Teachers have to go beyond traditional feelings that one can only read from books. Since an important goal is to create informed citizens, students should be encouraged to read and understand newspapers. Especially when first developing reading skills, many students feel overwhelmed at the prospect of reading a lengthy text. Short stories or magazine articles are more manageable and appealing.

In the third section of the survey students are asked to note the types of writing they prefer. You may find that as students complete the survey they note that they have never read or written some of the suggestions on the list and are unsure about responding to them. In this case, you might advise them to check those assignments that sound like fun and that they might like to try. Later, as they complete them, you can observe their level of enthusiasm to see their actual enjoyment. Of any of the choices on the list, many students seem to enjoy writing in a diary: yet, on first response, when diaries are described as containing personal information, most middle and high school students hesitate to select them because they do not want to share private thoughts and observations with teachers. Yet students who were

Figure 2-1. Student Interest Survey.

STUDENT INTEREST SURVEY
Karen A. Waldron, Ph.D.

NAME _____ DATE _____

TEACHER _____

GRADE _____

Directions: Everyone learns differently, and we want to find out how you learn the best. Please answer the following questions so we can help make school interesting and fun.

1. At school, what types of activities do you like the best? Please check each of your favorites.

READING AND WRITING

I like to READ and WRITE about:

_____ people		_____ sports
_____ adventure		_____ history
_____ space science fiction		_____ science
_____ hobbies		_____ things that have really happened

OTHER (please discuss) _____

_____

2. My favorite ways to READ things include:

_____ textbooks	_____ short stories
_____ library books	_____ poetry
_____ newspapers	_____ comics
_____ magazines	_____ plays

OTHER (please discuss) _____

3. I most like to WRITE:

_____ reports for class about my hobbies or opinions	_____ letters to friends
	_____ word games or crossword puzzles
_____ short stories	_____ diary or journal entries about my feelings
_____ poetry	
_____ newspaper articles	

OTHER (please discuss) _____

ARITHMETIC

4. In MATH, I really like

_____ word problems	_____ multiplication
_____ number problems	_____ division
_____ addition	_____ fractions
_____ subtraction	_____ decimals
	_____ percentages

OTHER (please discuss) _____

_____

(continued)

45

(continued)

5. My favorite ways to learn MATH include

_____ doing problems on worksheets

_____ using a calculator

_____ doing a budget to manage my money

_____ puzzles and logic games

_____ learning about the stock market

_____ math games on a computer

_____ store catalogues where I can practice ordering things

OTHER (please discuss) _____

_____

6. Please tell us the way that you learn things best in the classroom, so we will know what you like. MY BEST WAYS TO LEARN THINGS INCLUDE:

_____ working in a large group when the teacher explains information to everybody at the same time

_____ working in a group with 2 or 3 other students

_____ working with 1 other student

_____ working by myself

_____ finishing worksheets at my desk

_____ watching films, videotapes, and filmstrips

_____ working at the computer

_____ working at Learning Centers

_____ doing "Hand's On" things like experiments or cooking, where I get to see and touch things we're learning about

_____ when we take field trips where I get to see new places

_____ OTHER (please discuss)

_____

7. While tests are hard for everybody to take, sometimes one kind of test is easier for you. Please tell us the kind of test you prefer. I DO MY BEST ON TESTS WHEN:

_____ I read them myself and the teacher collects my paper at the same time as everyone else's.

_____ I have extra time to write my answers.

_____ The questions are not written so closely together.

_____ Someone reads the questions to me and I write down my answers.

_____ Someone reads the questions to me and I tell them the answer without writing it down.

_____ I hear the questions from a tape recorder and I answer into the tape recorder.

_____ I show you my daily classwork and that counts for my grade instead of the test.

8. Everyone has favorite things they like to do. Please share yours with us so we get to know you better.

WHEN I HAVE TIME ALONE OUTSIDE OF SCHOOL, I MOST ENJOY
_____
_____

WHEN I AM WITH MY FRIENDS, I MOST ENJOY _____
_____

THE SUBJECTS I LIKE MOST AT SCHOOL ARE _____
_____

almost "writing-phobic" have begun to write again when they feel that the written information would not be shared with anyone for criticism or response. Diaries can be used to motivate students to write, are best shared only at the suggestion of the student, and should not be used as a basis for correcting grammar, punctuation and spelling. However, once the student is motivated to write, teachers then can expand the expectations for syntax and style and use student stories and reports as teaching tools.

Arithmetic is different. In the survey, the fourth section asks students to note the types of math problems they most enjoy. Understandably, students usually check the ones they perform the best. Students with cognitive or reading disabilities rarely like word problems because of the comprehension and analysis skills required. In actual computation, students with learning disabilities usually have the most difficulty completing problems with fractions, decimals, and percentages—probably because of the sophistication of part-whole relationships.

Learning which math operations are easiest for students does not indicate how they most enjoy reinforcement. This selection list is in the fifth section of the survey. Usually, students are most familiar with reinforcement of math skills by worksheets and may not have performed some of these activities, such as studying the stock market or using store catalogues to "order" merchandise. Since these activities are fun for teachers as well as students, you might want to try them and see if you both enjoy math more. (Try to not be too despondent if the students' stocks perform much better than yours.)

The sixth section asks students to complete their learning preferences. These responses are invaluable for considering how to structure the teaching-learning that goes on in the classroom. Students know how they have learned best in the past, and it is easier to design classrooms when they note their preferences.

Section seven includes questions about taking tests. While most students would prefer not taking tests, they rarely are given this option within most grading systems; perhaps the last choice on the list, substituting daily work for exams comes closest. Most students with learning differences do require some test-taking modification and often check several preferences on the survey. Some of these alternatives can take place in the regular classroom while others clearly require support by specialists. This guide can provide a basis for preference consideration.

The questions in the eighth section of the survey are open-ended and allow students to write in activities preferences and hobbies that may not have been considered on previous questions. The last statement encourages an expression of what has happened in a classroom that makes the student enjoy the subject matter. Often, responses include "I like science because the teacher is really funny," reinforcing the need of this student for a positive attitude, or "I like recess best because I don't have to sit still anymore," noting the student's need for physical activities interspersed throughout the day. Teachers can learn so much from students when they ask them their preferences.

STEP 2: PRESENTING INSTRUCTIONAL INFORMATION TO STUDENTS

Clearly the next step is the most difficult. It involves using the information that the students provided on the survey to create a motivational learning environment. While learning cannot always be fun, if students are having a good time learning, the teacher usually is having a good time teaching.

Chapter 1 included discussion of the need to begin the year by examining student records and appraisal information and establishing goals for students based on their learning needs. Their needs now can be combined with their interests and a classroom established where information is presented in a variety of ways designed to meet their assessed learning styles. Mrs. Dixon is an auditory learner, so when she teaches, she talks. She does not understand that her learning style has worked for her but might not work for her students. If her students had a sensory loss such as deafness, Mrs. Dixon would know to change her teaching style to include more visual and tactile supports. But students with learning disabilities have needs that may differ in less obvious ways, yet which require the same degree of modification.

To teach to a variety of learning needs, teachers need first to consider the array of options available in presenting information to students. Traditionally, a lecture by the teacher and follow-up reading from the text or completion of worksheets have comprised instruction in most classrooms, especially at the secondary level. In many resource and Content Mastery classrooms, the structure is similar: the student does not understand something, so the teacher explains the information, provides reinforcement activities and moves on to the next student. But some students do not listen well, usually because they tend to be more visual in their learning style or because they have Attention Deficit Hyperactivity Disorder and are highly distracted by stimuli in the classroom such as other students' voices or other students walking about the room. Since their attention span usually is short, they may lose concentration during the teacher's explanation or during reinforcement activities.

When these students are actively involved in the activity instead of just trying to listen to the teacher, they usually are able to concentrate longer and to become less distracted by external stimuli. What types of activities compel their attention? A number of these were listed on the Student Activity Survey, but bear more intense consideration.

1. *Class Discussions.* While class discussions always have been a successful teaching technique, they have been used more frequently in general education than in special education. Teachers have not tried to exclude students with special needs from discussing their observations, but their learning needs often are so pronounced that it has been more expedient for the teacher to provide the explanation instead of "wasting time" waiting for students to discover the answers themselves. The teacher has a sense that the class can then move more quickly and cover more information.

An adolescent once tested for learning problems commented on a number of responses, "I was taught that—I learned that. I just can't remember the answer." Yet, teaching involves learning. If learning has not taken place, usually teaching has not taken place either.

Students with learning disabilities often enjoy class discussions if they are included. However, whether in regular or special education, students with more severe learning problems rarely participate, usually because of fear of failure based on previous mistakes. The best way to have students involved in large group discussions is to ask them questions that you are sure they can answer, so that they do not suffer embarrassment in front of their peers. Teachers can select these questions by ongoing observation of students' written work as well as by understanding their cognitive level: concrete and factual, capable of understanding main ideas, or able to deal with abstractions. This information comes from observing students' verbal responses in other classroom situations.

Students rarely consider whether the questions they answer in class are difficult or easy, but they do attend to whether they have answered correctly and if the teacher response to their answer is positive or negative. The way teachers respond to student comments sets the stage for students' willingness to respond in the future. If the answer is wrong, it is important to rephrase the question and at times to give the student more supportive information so that the answer can be corrected. If the question was too difficult and no rephrasing will help, the teacher might quietly ask, "Would you like some help with that answer?" Rarely will you find a student who refuses.

Once students are confident that you will respond positively to any effort on their part, whether they get the answer or not, they tend to risk participation in the future, even when they are less sure about the correctness of their response. They will have learned to trust you.

Another type of class discussion is conducted by the students, not the teacher, and takes place in small groups. Again, structure is the key, especially when students may be disorganized and tend to have problems following directions. While specific grouping methods will be discussed, it is important for teachers to realize that almost any small grouping arrangement can be successful if students' expected outcomes are carefully discussed in advance.

For example, students in resource, Content Mastery, and regular education classrooms can be placed together in homogeneous or heterogeneous groups in any content area after they have read a passage in a text, received instruction in how to compute a math problem, or been given an activity in logical problem-solving. The group runs best when given written directions about questions they are to answer and told in advance how much time they have to complete the assignments. When members are assigned specific roles within the group, small groups containing three or four students are optimal. The teacher should walk around the room as the students are answering the questions, redirecting anyone off-task and being sure that students understand the directions.

When students are grouped heterogeneously, the more academically capable students may tend to answer all the questions. To help avoid this, quieter nonparticipants can be asked questions by the teacher to encourage their responsiveness. Additionally, many of the students with more extensive learning problems do gain in their understanding of the material based on listening to their peers' explanations. Many times students discuss ideas most successfully with each other.

After the small groups meet, the teacher should allow at least 10 minutes at the end of the class for large group discussion. During this time, the teacher asks each group to respond to the specified questions. The more basic questions can be directed to the students with concrete learning styles (i.e., "Where did Mark go when he left home?"), and the more conceptual questions to students with higher abstraction skills (i.e., "Although he said he was mad at his father, what do you think was the *real* reason Mark ran away?") In this way, all students can participate in both small and large group discussions and feel good about their involvement.

Barbara comments, "I can see where these small group arrangements would work well for some of my students, but I also can see students like Sean and Marcus fooling around and not paying a bit of attention during groupwork. They do it now during large group discussions and I'm sure they would ruin the small groups as well." You may be right, Barbara. Some students cannot participate in group discussions because they do not have a long enough attention span or because of poor behaviors. But these students tend to do best in "hands-on" activities directed toward their interests.

2. *Participatory Learning.* The principle of "mutual exclusion" often works well with students with learning differences. They cannot be hitting someone while they are concentrating on a writing task; they cannot be calling across the room if they are engrossed in reading their part in a play. Traditionally, teachers have believed that they must give students information by telling them what they need to know. Yet students with special needs learn best if they are actively involved in the lesson as it develops.

Sam was a highly anxious adolescent, small for his age, gifted, but with a learning disability in verbal and written expressive language. He was enrolled in regular and honors high school classes, and while he did not "officially" attend special education, the resource teacher consulted with his teachers weekly to give support and suggestions to improve his performance.

Although he was highly conceptual, Sam could not organize his thoughts well and avoided all speaking and writing tasks. While he could be motivated to at least attempt written assignments, Sam could not be persuaded to answer questions or to verbally participate in class. Even when he clearly knew the answer, if called upon, Sam's face would turn scarlet, his body would visibly shake, and he would hang his head, unable to speak. He was the quietest person his teachers had ever known.

Based on the idea of participatory learning, Sam's English teacher decided that he did not need lectures or even class discussions where everyone else talked. He definitely needed situations where he was comfortable explaining ideas to someone else. One afternoon, Sam's arrival at the school Chess Club, which was sponsored by the English teacher, provided the direction. He was comfortable there, with about ten games running simultaneously, intelligent people conceptualizing, and above all, no need to talk. He also was good at chess and managed to win often. With the belief that guidance counselors really like to guide and counsel more than to schedule students into classes, the teacher turned to Mr. Grady for help. He was a kind, interactive, and importantly, nonthreatening man who cared about students. He was a novice chess player and had visited the club a few times to observe the players. One afternoon the teacher discussed Sam's communication problems with him and suggested that Sam might become a chess teacher for Mr. Grady, allowing Sam the opportunity to discuss moves as the need arose, but to be involved with a nonthreatening adult in a quiet setting. Mr. Grady was very enthused, the next day asked Sam to teach him chess, and Sam was far too nonverbal to refuse.

Starting the following Friday, Sam went to Mr. Grady's small office during English period when the rest of the class had their "free-reading" day. Mr. Grady reported that in the safety of this environment, Sam was willing to offer terse directions on moving chess pieces and, over time, even on chess strategies. They continued their relationship until Sam graduated high school; when Sam moved up into other high school classes where he could not be released during the school day, they began playing weekly after school. At Mr. Grady's suggestion, they often played during Chess Club meetings, where Sam eventually was selected as the instructor for student novices entering the group. He was extremely proud of this role, and of course, had to talk with the students as he explained the game.

While Sam likely never became an orator, being an active participant was the key to meeting both his psychological and learning needs. Although most students are not as difficult to involve as Sam, when passive students are involved, they learn better. Resource and Content Mastery teachers have a tendency to believe that their role is set for them by others, usually because of logistical reasons such as scheduling. Yet in their rooms, they can be as creative and involve students as much as they want without being forced into the traditional lecturer role.

Additional "hands-on" activities can be as innovative and creative as the educator. Although your school views Content Mastery as a support for the regular classroom, this does not mean that the only instruction should involve rote learning. For example, if several students come to you having problems reading a play (anything from *Flowers for Algernon* to *Julius Caesar*) you might assign roles among students, have them read the lines aloud and discuss the play's meaning. Or when certain students are assigned to your resource room for reading, arithmetic or listening comprehension problems, you might enjoy following recipes and cooking or baking delicacies.

In Alamo Heights Independent School District, San Antonio, Texas, a few of the resource teachers combine their classes each class period on Friday and have a theme day where students study the art, history, and social customs of another country. If they cannot finish all the information in one day, they continue studying it the next Friday. To be able to participate each week, resource students bring a behavioral checklist completed by their regular classroom teachers, indicating that they have shown strong effort during the week and have completed all assigned work. Fridays are so exciting for the resource students that they rarely bring negative reports. And teachers involved tell how the regular education students not enrolled in the resource program drop in all day, eager to hear music and taste different foods. This student responsiveness certainly has taken much of the stigma away from special class attendance since the nonenrolled students ask why they cannot attend also.

3. *Field-visits (Bringing the Field to the Classroom).* An extension of the participatory learning method is having the students observe and learn from what others outside the school are doing. While resource students should have additional opportunities to visit community locations, unfortunately this is rarely the case. Often justifiably, regular education teachers complain about students missing work in their classes.

But it can be more functional to have visitors come to the school to discuss with students or to demonstrate what they do. For example, parents or community members might demonstrate how they design and paint, or sculpt, for their profession or hobby. A mechanic may discuss with high school students things they can look for and do when they are having car trouble. Or a member of the police or traffic department could give a series of mini-lessons on defensive driving. A banker could discuss obtaining financial credit and emphasize what to avoid in overspending. A musician from the local symphony could demonstrate and explain different types of musical instruments, or a nurse could discuss how to prevent hearing loss when attending "rock" concerts. One young student became extremely enthused when, on Beethoven's birthday, the teacher played several Beethoven compositions and discussed the artist's life. The child excitedly reported to his parents, "He wrote all that pretty music and he couldn't even hear it! He was *death!*" His parents provided a bit more instruction.

The possibilities for classroom visitors and/or demonstration are endless. When scheduling is a problem because a visitor cannot stay all day and students attend at a variety of times, the demonstration and discussion might be held before school for everyone, with parents invited, or during the lunch hour(s), when students are asked to bring a sack lunch. Often, many students outside special education want to attend these sessions, again adding credibility to teacher efforts.

4. *Media.* As educators reconceptualize their sense of what should be happening in resource and Content Mastery classes they must understand the wonderful support available from instructional media. Media are not just films that regular classroom teachers occasionally show. Media use is a way of providing information through a variety of learning modalities, allowing children with special needs to gain new information or reinforcement through a number of channels, not just lectures or reading.

In the model Content Mastery program in Carrollton-Farmers Branch Independent School District, teachers' rooms are laden with media and materials. Many teachers have an audiotape of every book their students use in regular education. Each book is divided into chapters on the tape, and a student with a reading problem comes to the room and reads the text with the tape accompaniment. This support alone has allowed numerous students to continue their participation in the regular classroom. While most teachers do not have the time to tape their books, a classroom teaching assistant, a parent, or an older student who is a proficient reader can do so. And as the American Printing House for the Blind extends its supports to students with visual-perceptual disorders, with advance notice these books can be ordered and kept in the resource room.

More videotapes are being created to include "smart-talk" for students experiencing social problems with peers or difficulties with parents and teachers. These tapes could be shown on a specified day, or students could view them when their academic work is completed, leaving time for discussion. Other areas, such as reading by phonics, classroom organizational skills, and applying for a job, can be taught with the support of materials packages, many of which contain media and reinforcement activities.

These resources are available through the Regional Service Centers and the Instructional Media Centers in school districts. Teachers usually can borrow a few at a time for several weeks. If the teacher visits the regional or school center in August before school starts and makes a list of pertinent materials, the school counselor or librarian can order them as the teacher needs them without the the inconvenience of a return trip to the center. Several teachers in related subject areas can combine materials and media to have a larger store to use with varied teacher needs. The consulting teacher also can loan materials to the regular classroom teacher or can note which specific materials or media this teacher might want to borrow directly to support a particular student's learning style.

5. *Content-Based Units.* It was disappointing to hear a first-year teacher from a reputable teacher-training program note that "We don't believe in unit-instruction anymore." Unfortunately, the new trends in redesigning instructional management may be neglecting one of the most motivational of teaching strategies: finding a content area of student interest and exploring it intensively to teach basic skills and add new knowledge.

A regular education teacher interested in a number of native Indian tribes that had settled local regions was determined to expand student knowledge despite their lack of interest. Her pupils "became" Iroquois and Algonquian Indians: they built teepees, followed the laws of the land, and shared common foods. They led tribal meetings, staged wars, and settled disputes within their boundaries. Previously disinterested students began appearing in the classroom before school started, claiming that at home the night before they had re-thought decisions made during the tribal council and wished they had voted differently. They began to compare their involvements with those of modern governments, finding tremendous parallels and differences. It was exciting, and students became motivated and knowledgeable.

Barbara interjects, "But I'm usually called on to be a remedial specialist, or worse, a tutor. When teachers send me purple ditto sheets that I'm supposed to use in reinforcing what they're teaching in class, how can I do unit instruction? We're lucky to get those sheets finished with the students even partially understanding the content."

Within that structure, Barbara, you can only become frustrated and "burn-out." The key will be to re-define the role of classes for students with special needs so that you do provide support, but so that you also are allowed to creatively teach students concepts that they do not understand. A wonderful high school teacher in a resource class watched her students fall further behind in their regular English class as they were forced to read *Julius Caesar.* They were as bored in her room reading the play as they had been in their regular class. At first she made the common mistake of trying to teach the information in the same way that it was taught in their classes. Then, after several

days of frustration, she realized that if the students could understand it when it was taught in regular education, they would not
be coming to her. She immediately changed to a more creative
approach, with students spending part of each resource session
building a model Globe Theater, discussing modern politicians
who might be like the characters in the play, and interpreting
meaning through acting. Her results were so "dramatic" and the
students so enthused that a number of regular education
teachers borrowed her ideas to use in their classes.

Most schools do not dictate how to reinforce learning in
special units, but view the individual classroom as the teacher's
personal area of expertise. Avoid the tendency to feel that you
cannot be innovative, that the system will not allow you to do
more than rote repetition of regular classroom teaching. Most
administrators are delighted when parents indicate that their
child has become excited about school because of a motivational teacher.

6. *Academic Clubs.* No setting can better capture this sense
of excitement about learning than "The Lab School," in Washington, DC. Directed by Dr. Sally Smith, this school relies primarily on an extension of unit teaching and participatory learning called "Academic Clubs," which provide ongoing motivation
and involvement by students.

These "clubs" (the word itself implying membership and
belonging within a group) are based on an environmental approach to teaching. Students are immersed daily in a setting
totally directed toward mythology ("Gods' Club"), the Renais-
sance, philosophy, a period of American history ("Pioneers'
Club") or literature ("Charles Dickens' Club"), or any area of
general student interest, such as the "Secret Agents' Club" for
reading readiness skills, the "Broadcasters' Club" for language
development, or the "Pirates' Club" for studying maps,
directionality, and distances.

As students enter the room, they change their name, role,
and time or location to join a different aspect of history, literature, or society. Largely based on teaching through the arts,
students don simple costumes and begin work on the project of
the day, which may emphasize any instructional area, based on
the direction of the teacher, who assumes the leadership role
appropriate to the setting. Students in one room may be completing a model railroad with cars stopping at the different lo-

cations of Civil War battles. Another room can be turned into a cave, with students developing a written symbolic language which could indicate concerns of early human existence. The sense of cooperation and cameraderie is wonderful as students purposefully move about the room.

While Barbara may not be convinced to don a toga and begin teaching Roman History, it is important to note that "Academic Clubs" discourage discipline problems. The structure and motivation is such that students want to participate and to belong to the clubs. Again, mutual exclusion. They cannot be fighting with someone at the same time they are designing "to-scale" maps in their cartography club.

What is the possibility of including this in-depth immersion strategy in resource and Content Mastery classes? Again, educators are limited only by the extent of imagination. In an earlier example of participatory learning, two resource teachers were combining their classes on Fridays to immerse students in different cultures. They continued their "Fun Friday" program all day; they differed the activities at any one time based on the needs and capability levels of the students in third period versus fifth period. They could emphasize literature, or history, or music, or foods as a topic during the day, but vary the content for appropriateness.

The topics are endless and exciting. Teachers in The Lab School have found it necessary to research certain areas with which they are not as familiar, but they note that it is also fun for them to learn new things and to share this information with their students. Once they formulate a good "Academic Club," they save their information and plans and use them again.

7. *Learning Centers.* Teachers also can have variety within their daily classrooms without relying on immersion as a total philosophy. Clues here come from regular education, where elementary school teachers have had learning centers for a number of years as a means of meeting individual student needs within large-group structures. But learning centers need not only be used in regular or elementary classrooms. Their purposes are ideal for specialized settings at elementary and secondary levels.

Centers underscore the concept of variety within student learning needs, styles, and content by providing the ability to teach or reinforce skills at individual rates and levels. For example, each room might have a listening center, where students could listen to tapes of individual books being read in regular classes. There could be an arithmetic center with concrete objects, such a cuisennaire rods, to support student skill-building. A high school room could include kits with high interest-low vocabulary books and materials dealing with topics in history, English, or science, adding reinforcement to regular classroom instruction. As noted previously, materials for many of the centers can be borrowed from Regional Service Centers or District Centers.

Since reading is primarily social in its motivation (Elkind, 1988), it is important to provide students a comfortable place where they can read materials from their regular classes as well as additional books and magazines. While the location needs to be in a quiet area of the classroom to avoid distractions, it also should be pleasant and relaxing. Many teachers have a colorful carpet on which students can read or even a loft area with a positive atmosphere. Chapter 5 will include discussion of how students can independently use the centers while the teacher serves as a resource.

8. *Computers.* Although computers are seen as a luxury in many schools, they can be invaluable for students with learning disabilities. While they cannot easily take the place of a teacher's direct instruction, they can supply reinforcement for many instructional areas. For example, in using the computer for skills support, students can be allowed all the time they need to learn a concept, to think about the meaning of a reading passage, or to consider a math problem, quite unlike traditional classroom instruction, where the teacher moves along far too rapidly for many students. As Lerner (1988) points out, computers are also private. Students do not make mistakes publicly and suffer embarrassment: computers are truly "friendly," unlike a more judgmental classmate, and usually offer nothing harsher than a quiet "Try again."

Many computer educational games force the reader to respond automatically, building fluency in reading sight words, performing basic math computations, or increasing spelling vocabulary. The variety of word processing software now available makes the teaching of written expression far easier since students can correct errors and revise their text without much effort. Dysgraphic students lose the stigma of indecipherable handwriting, there is no longer a concern about having to "rewrite" the entire text if changes are made, and the review of written material during proofreading is so much easier. Enticing innovations such as LOGO (Cosden & Semmel, 1987) motivate students through graphics use while they learn and reinforce concepts in a variety of areas, such as problem-solving skills and basic elements of programming.

Mark was a fifth-grade student diagnosed both as learning disabled and gifted. While he was in regular education for most of his instruction, he attended one period of resource daily and was part of a weekly "pull-out" program for gifted students. While he loved participating in the gifted program, he hated attending the traditional resource room, mainly because of the stigma he felt from his gifted peers. He eventually refused to attend the resource class, and when forced, became aggressive and disruptive.

A collaborative model was used to support Mark's success in regular education, removing him from any attendance in the resource room. However, since the team did not want him to feel that he had won through aggression, he was required to sign a contract that in the regular classroom he would voluntarily complete all reinforcement work in written expression, his area of disability. Each Friday, the resource teacher met with his regular classroom teacher, reviewed his week's work and offered suggestions for handling any problems that had arisen. She also provided materials and reinforcement strategies.

Despite these collaborative efforts and the use of contracting, the recurring problem was his avoidance of written work, marked by his overly hasty performance or total refusal. Consultation with his teacher in the gifted class indicated that Mark always asked to use the computer and that she had to make him share it with other students. The way to his heart was clearly there.

Mark's regular classroom teacher worked a schedule with the teacher of the gifted class so that when the "gifted room" was free, he could use the computer to complete his written work. The results were outstanding and immediate. Mark was required to write a rough draft of most work by hand (in case a computer would not always be available to him), but he could write all final copies on the computer. Not only did he complete his work quickly and excitedly, but he became "hooked" on computers in the way gifted students often do. By the end of the year, school district administrators published two computer programs Mark had written about local history, and presented him with an academic achievement award. He was the only student in 93 schools to receive this particular award, and none of the judges knew he had a learning disability. Computers can make a difference in motivation as well as reinforcement.

STEP 3: VARYING CONTENT PRESENTATION ACCORDING TO STUDENT NEEDS

Laurie, Buchwach, Silverman, and Zigmond (1978) note several variables with which teachers must be concerned to meet student needs through the previously discussed methods: the *conceptual level* of students, the *amount of information* they can learn at any one period, and the *amount of time* they require to complete a task. Teachers who have worked with students with learning disabilities understand that conceptual abilities can vary tremendously. Clearly this spectrum of students cannot be taught the same way. Mark, the computer expert, was motivated through an "interest binge" so typical of gifted students. But that was Mark. Another student might be able to best use the computer for reinforcement of math or spelling, but not have the conceptual abilities to explore advanced software demands or, certainly, to be involved in programming.

Previous discussion noted how students with learning differences often have short attention spans and are so easily distracted that concentration is eroded. They simply cannot handle the same amount of information as students with longer attention spans. For these students, briefer assignments with frequent breaks work best to sustain their on-task behaviors. Teachers often are surprised at the amount of work students can accomplish when they use suggestions discussed in Chapter I, such as a less distractible environment and a limitation of the number of instructional variables.

Additionally, students often require different amounts of time to complete the same assignment. In this way, students with special needs are no different than students in general education. For example, any third- or tenth-grade teacher knows that the traditional practice of collecting class assignments after 20 minutes of work results in some students finishing early, wasting their time and creating a potential disturbance, others not being able to finish although they know the information and could do quite well with additional time. Often students are tested for the time it takes them to complete a task instead of for their content knowledge. In special education units, where students often have more extreme variations in learning styles and in time requirements for task completion, assignments should be shortened for certain students if the teacher faces time constraints, or students should be allowed as much time as they need.

These three variables of amount of information students can digest, its conceptual level, and time required for task completion should be treated as an integral aspect of selection among the methods of presentation discussed in Step 2. For example, a student with a short attention span and a comparatively lower ability to handle abstractions is more likely to be successful when taught through learning centers, unit activities, and "Academic Clubs," since these approaches involve exploratory learning, are usually best at motivating students, and allow for more movement during learning than do desk activities. A student can more easily take a break for a minute or two, get a drink of water, and return to a learning center than to a formal large-group activity, or even a computer. On the other hand, a student with higher conceptual skills and time-on-task abilities might enjoy computer work or attending to visitors talking to the group or working as a leader in a small-group task such as writing for the class newsletter. Choice of instructional method always should be based on observations of student learning styles and needs, and a variety of these approaches in any one room allows a greater deal of flexibility in planning for students.

Barbara interjects, "Although I won't be able to create all these instructional changes at once, there are certain ones that I think the students might enjoy and I would find creative. But what about my discipline problems? I can see where Sean would interrupt visitors as they spoke and might destroy materials in the learning centers. What can I do about him?"

You're right, Barbara. An instructional framework of varied teaching methods cannot work if students are not in control of their behaviors. Chapters 3 and 4 will include discussion of behavior management strategies. However, you have already started to affect student behaviors when you implement the changes discussed in this chapter, because you have looked at students' individual motivational and learning needs and are selecting those most suited to a student's ability to attend to task. By the "mutual exclusion" principle, Sean will not rush to destroy materials in a learning center if he finds that using them is fun.

SUMMARY

Discussion in this chapter emphasized the need for student-centered classrooms where teachers set the direction and select instruction based on individual student learning styles. More recent instructional models for service delivery, such as Content Mastery, were reviewed, with the conclusion that these programs can be excellent in developing skills in some students, but there is no single method that is effective with everyone. For example, it does not appear to be more important whether a student is in a Content Mastery unit or a resource classroom: what matters is the setting of realistic, attainable student goals, developing the best teaching methods to accomplish these goals, and motivating students so they will want to learn, through personal commitment to the goals and activities.

A Student Interest Survey was reviewed as a basis for discovering how students prefer to learn and teaching strategies they have personally enjoyed in the past. A broad array of areas can be explored in this survey, from formats in reading, written expression, and arithmetic to the types of testing arrangements students have found most successful. An example of a survey was provided, and teachers were encouraged to adapt it to their own needs.

As Barbara quickly noted, such a variety of choices requires a broad number of ways of presenting instructional information within the classroom. Nine separate ways of encouraging learning were included. The tenth way, large-group instruction, was purposefully omitted as a primary teaching method, since students with special needs rarely succeed by this method and its common use in regular education classrooms is often the reason students initially are placed in special education. Within this variety of methods were included everything from small-group work and participatory activities to including guest speakers, using media, and developing learning centers. Additional suggestions involved unit study based on motivational content, extending at times to Academic Clubs, where students are immersed in a setting or time period to allow for improved understanding. Potential uses for computers as content reinforcers or word processors were noted, as well as their providing a basis for gifted students to use sophisticated software.

Despite the instructional methods used, the importance of varying content presentation according to student needs was underscored. Close observation of students' conceptual level, the amount of information they can digest within a lesson, and the time they require for task completion are critical variables for selecting the best teaching methods. Since even a motivational, appropriate method may lose its impact if used too often, teachers are encouraged to use variety in their teaching, keeping their own motivation high.

Chapter 3 includes discussion of how to develop a personalized discipline plan so that managing student behaviors can be as successful as developing teaching strategies.

Chapter 3

MANAGING STUDENT BEHAVIORS

Behavior problems may hinder learning more than an actual learning disability. As discussed in Chapter 2, although providing work directed toward student interests and varying methods of presenting information in the classroom will prevent the occurrence of many student behavior problems, there are still students who will misbehave. As a veteran teacher, Barbara might provide a list of those student behaviors that interfere most often with the teaching-learning process.

"I'd be delighted, since I'm totally frustrated in the behavior management area. Types of student behavior problems tend to fall into one of several categories: the disruptive category seems never-ending, with students off-task, talking or just fooling around; then, from others are the aggressive, impulse-directed outbursts, or the opposite, apathetic, nonparticipation. While aggressive students always demand my immediate attention and often interrupt others' learning, I find apathetic students to be more exasperating because their total lack of interest and involvement makes me feel like a poor teacher since I can't reach them."

Before discussing the specific behaviors of students in these categories, teacher sensitivity to student responses should be considered. Children, and especially adolescents, misbehave for a variety of reasons, many of which have nothing to do with the teacher or class. Their words or actions cannot be taken personally. If you have ever noted how slowly many students board the bus home on Friday afternoon, or have watched how long it takes them to change back from their high-strung Monday morning actions to more even, relaxed responses after a few hours in school, you will realize that *school itself is rarely the cause of the inappropriate behaviors these students demonstrate.* As a matter of fact, school may be the only constant in some of these young people's lives, and actually teachers may be their model of consistency and caring. The fact that Barbara feels frustrated means that she cares, and this deep caring is evident in progressively more teachers as societal problems increase. While positive ways of working with the family will be discussed in Chapter 6, it is important that teachers never negate themselves or their efforts when dealing with difficult-to-manage students.

Although it is clearly advisable to stay as objective as possible when working with students, teachers are human and do react emotionally at times. The second suggestion is to allow yourself to realize how frustrating the behavior of some students can be, and *if you become angry at all, your anger should be directed at the behavior and not at the student.* If students speak rudely, you can allow yourself to think badly of their family, their manners and themselves as individuals, feeding your anger, or you can realize that the students have a behavior which needs changing and not reject them personally because of misdirected anger. Taking blame away from the student and responding to the behavior enables educators to become more objective and clearheaded in their response.

Another general consideration is always to respond to the behaviors of individual students and not to generalize consequences to the group, many of whose members may not have been involved at all. Most people can recall times in elementary school where a few students misbehaved and the entire class was kept from recess, or in high school where one or two students did not complete their homework and the teacher penalized the class by giving everyone an additional assignment. These occasions are remembered because they were not fair: consequences should have been administered to students whose behaviors were unacceptable, not to the entire group because the teacher was angry or upset. Students are very observant about "fairness" and become upset easily when they are punished for others' misbehaviors. Teachers who react to the group instead of the individual often create the negative climate discussed earlier, one which is counterproductive to learning.

But what are the behaviors teachers find the most difficult? Figure 3-1 lists them by Barbara's categories: those that are disruptive, or verbally and physically aggressive, or those that are noninvolved and apathetic. While teachers tend to focus on the aggression, off-task, disruptive behaviors actually are more pervasive (Jones, 1987), especially in classrooms where students with Attention Deficit Hyperactivity Disorder may predominate. Seemingly driven by lack of impulse control and distractibility, these students talk to others at will, at times calling across the room, completely disturbing the teacher and the class. When others are speaking, these students interrupt without thought. Those who are hyperactive leave their seats without permission, wander around the classroom completely oblivious to instruction. They may begin "clowning around" with others innocently, until they distract other students from their work, knock books on the floor, or generally make it impossible to teach.

The aggressive students tend to behave disruptively in class, interfering with their own learning and that of other students. These students can be rude and defiant, at times verbally or

---

DISRUPTIVE (IMPULSE DRIVEN)

Calling out
Out-of-seat
Talking with others
"Clowning around"
Throwing things

APATHETIC

Not completing class
    assignments independently
Not completing homework
Lack of concern about grades
Nonparticipation in large and
    small group activities
Nonresponsive to highly
    motivational activities

AGGRESSIVE

Rudeness to others
Physical aggression
Defiant when asked to follow rules
Fighting

DISORGANIZED

Loses class materials, papers
Loses homework
Does not record assignments
    correctly
Difficulty following directions
Overall sense of confusion
Difficulty with transitions between
    assignments and groups
Difficulty transferring between
    concepts

Figure 3-1. Common behavior problems of students with learning differences.

even physically attacking the teacher or other students. They angrily refuse to do as they are told and favor confrontation over cooperation. They often mock class rules and have a "Make me do it!" attitude, demonstrating a general disregard for classroom rules or the rights of others.

As Barbara will attest, it is impossible to teach in a classroom when students are out of their seats, fighting with others and responding defiantly to teachers as they try to regain order. No one likes to be treated rudely, and certainly no one likes to feel personal physical threats from students. Discipline failures with unruly students are a primary reason why even the most devoted, caring teachers burn out and leave the profession.

Recently, an example of this was evidenced in a self-contained classroom for children with severe learning problems, where the teacher was a veteran of many years. Although her students learned slowly and needed much intervention, she loved them and took pleasure as they expanded their skills. But this year the district placed a student with severely disruptive and aggressive behaviors in her class. Out of control, the student was physically threatening to others in class, including the teacher and teacher-assistant. No one felt safe. When the teacher requested that the student be removed from her class and placed in a class for the emotionally disturbed, she was told that the unit was full and that since the student had learning as well as behavioral problems, she was eligible to remain in this classroom. Realizing that the student also would be in the class at least one more year, the teacher has applied for early retirement.

This story underscores what so many teachers have experienced. While it is often said, "A teacher can make a difference," it is all too obvious that a student can also make a difference—unfortunately, for the negative as well as the positive. The reasons for inappropriate, often aggressive behaviors must be understood first and then a plan developed for eliminating them.

Although the type of aggressiveness may vary, such behaviors usually are based on student impulsivity or expression of anger, and sometimes on both of these factors. While it never pays to "understand too much" (Elkind, 1989), some children are from homes where aggressive, acting-out behaviors are the norm, and they may be modeling what they see. Or they may have feelings of anger based on abuse, neglect, or difficult social and economic circumstances.

While teachers often comment that they could use a few more of the quiet, apathetic students in their classes, they eventually find that these students also are very disruptive to the learning environment. "I agree," notes Barbara. "I'm thinking of Kathy, a student I once taught. She was quiet, sweet, and certainly no one whom you would consider to be a behavior problem—until you walked away from her desk. Then she stopped all work, looked around the classroom and watched life go by. She completed no assignments unless given full teacher attention, and she certainly never did homework. She was a nondisruptive group member, but she just looked around, talked to no one, and usually did nothing more than scribble on a notepad. When I sent papers home, she lost them. When she was supposed to bring books or materials to class, she never had them and noncommitedly would say that she didn't know where they were. That was Kathy's problem: she was not committed to me, learning, her classmates, grades, anything. She just didn't care. Behavior problems such as hers can make teaching really difficult."

Barbara is expressing what many teachers feel. But the desire to return to the times when students listened, followed directions, and did their homework will not necessarily take educators back to that era. Students are different today. Even those who are not considered to have discipline problems voice their opinions more and are much more assertive around adults than children were years ago. Yet, teachers do not have to accept rudeness or lack of respect from any student. The first thing to do is analyze each teacher's personal needs in the classroom. Then a program can be designed to meet them.

ESTABLISHING PERSONAL NEEDS

While teachers today are as angry as many of their students, ironically they often feel that they do not have any rights to have their own personal and professional needs met. Yet, as discussed in Chapter 1, successful teachers possess positive attitudes, and these attitudes are based largely on the teacher's support by students, colleagues, administrators, and parents. Part of the current sense of teacher distress may be based on the community expecting the educational system to take over and "cure" numerous social problems. Many teachers have felt themselves treated as scapegoats for an inability to stem mammoth problems such as drug abuse. Yet, at the same time, their failure to raise standardized test scores has been criticized broadly.

In the face of these almost insoluable difficulties, teachers often feel they would receive a disbelieving reception if they were to state loudly that their own needs are not being met. Yet, until teachers take direction in shaping their own daily environment, the system will not change.

The individual classroom is the easiest place to begin this change. When teachers meet their students for the first time, they should discuss their expectations of student behaviors in the classroom. If your students sense that you do not expect very much of them, they will live up to your expectations. If you initially clarify your expectations for their behavior and consistently follow through with appropriate consequences for positive and negative behaviors, the students will integrate your expectations and begin to set higher expectations for their own and others' behaviors.

In a large, modern high school, teachers and students all smiled at the mention of "Mrs. Murray's" name. A veteran of more than 30 years of teaching high school, she had never changed her expectations for appropriate student behavior. As students entered her room, they were all expected to greet her cordially. They were to go immediately to their seats and take out their books or planned work for the day. When another adult entered the room, the entire class was to stand in acknowledgment of their respect for the adult role. As chauvanistic as it might first appear, if a female student left the room and returned, the closest male student was to stand up from his desk and acknowledge her. On the other hand the young woman was to smile and thank him, and she was to always be polite and interactive. The students all addressed Mrs. Murray by her name and said "Ma'am" when answering her. Without exception. No exceptions were allowed because Mrs. Murray assumed that all of her students were capable of mutual respect. At the beginning of the year, when a few "untrained" students responded sarcastically or did not follow her rules, they sat in time-out to consider them. The training worked.

But there was an additional attitude that made students respond to Mrs. Murray's eccentric demands. She always respected students. As they greeted her on entering the room, she asked about their families, admired their attire, or said how she had missed them during a recent school absence. And no one doubted that she had indeed missed them. They addressed her politely, and she called them "Mr." or "Miss" with their last name. (While students laughed at this at first, no one doubted that she was respecting them as people.) She never yelled or scolded when homework or schoolwork was not completed. She took the student aside, to prevent embarrassment, and spoke of her disappointment with his or her behavior. She quietly added a zero into the daily average so everyone knew she meant business. The students loved Mrs. Murray and competed to be in her class. Within the novelty of old-fashioned behaviors and demands, students flourished.

Of course there were students who added to her gray hairs. But the majority asked Mrs. Murray quietly, "What do you expect of me?" and she told them. They worked together in mutual respect. Mrs. Murray's story underscores that it is not the rules themselves that are important, but that behavioral guidelines are established in the classroom and that students know they are responsible for following them.

ESTABLISHING REQUIREMENTS FOR STUDENT BEHAVIOR

The questions in Figure 3-2 will allow teachers to consider what their own basic needs and preferences are in guiding student behaviors. Teachers should answer these questions before school begins, so they will know which behaviors to emphasize or eliminate. In answer to the first question, teachers should specifically note positive student behaviors that they enjoy instead of focusing on the negative. These might include simple interactive needs, such as politeness to the teacher and other students, or listening as others' speak. Additionally, basic to a successful learning environment, needs such as students' staying in their seats, raising hands, and performing work willingly are important to most teachers. None of these are shocking, all traditionally were understood, and yet today, many teachers have difficulty articulating them or requiring students to follow them.

As Redl and Wattenberg (1951) indicate, students today have their needs too. As you answer the first three questions in

---

DIRECTIONS: Please answer each of the following questions, carefully considering the type of classroom environment which would please you the most.

1. To derive pleasure from teaching in your classroom each day, what specific behaviors do you need for students to exhibit? (For example, listening to you and to other students; staying in their seats.)
2. What behaviors in the classroom do you see as most detrimental to the learning of all students in the class?
3. What behaviors in the classroom do you see as most detrimental to the learning of the individual student?
4. Which student behaviors make you feel the most overwhelmed and as if the class is out of control?
5. How do you give in-class assignments to students?
6. After completion of their assignments, how do students know what to do next?
7. What are the rules for appropriate behavior in the classroom?
8. What is the consequence for following or not following the rules?
9. How are grades assigned?
10. Do rules and the assignment of grades apply equally to all students in your class?

Figure 3-2. Questions for teachers to consider when establishing behavioral rules in the classroom. Adapted from Laurie et al. (1978). Teaching secondary learning disabled students in the mainstream. *Learning Disabilities Quarterly, 1,* 62-71.

Figure 3-2, ask students to consider them as well. For example, on the first day of school, you might tell students the positive behaviors you need to observe in class, and then ask which behaviors they would add to the list to support a positive learning environment. Similarly, you might note the behaviors they feel are most conducive for their concentration and optimal performance, and those behaviors that detract the most from their learning.

It can be surprising to note the strength of opinions younger students have about classroom rules that support their learning. Understanding their own degree of distractibility, they may note that talking by others, and even the sound of pencils writing, bother them. The rules that they establish for their behavior are far stricter than those you might establish for them.

Questions 5 to 10 focus on daily methods of conducting class which influence student behaviors, but which are areas that teachers often do not consider important. For example, if you verbally give directions for an in-class assignment, some students with auditory processing disabilities or memory problems may not follow the directions easily. If you write them on the board as well as say them, many more students may respond appropriately.

Question 6 includes consideration of "dead," or transition, time, when the task is completed and students need to proceed to the next assignment. While teachers rarely consider how to structure this time in advance, if no structure is provided discipline problems often occur during this period. Since variations in learning styles often cause students to complete assignments at different times, they should be directed by the teacher in what they are to do as others finish their work. In Chapter 5, a variety of ways to encourage constant time-on-task for students will be discussed, allowing them to move smoothly from one task to another.

Questions 7 and 8 are very important to an effective teaching-learning environment. The actual classroom rules are a result of consideration of the previous six questions. The rules should be stated directly, taking into account those behaviors you and the students have agreed are important. Stating the rules positively supports the sense of a positive setting. For example, you might include "Listen while others are talking," instead of "Don't talk while others are speaking."

It is important to be specific in rules statements, not using broad terms such as "good behavior," which may not indicate exactly what the student is to do. *Students with special needs learn very little incidentally.* They need to be told exactly what is expected of them.

While teachers would like students to behave well out of respect for the classroom environment, stimulating teaching, or interest in learning, this rarely happens. Students select their behaviors based on the consequences. Therefore, a direct statement of consequences for a particular behavior is particularly important. Positive consequences are more conducive to a cooperative environment. Teachers should avoid the pitfall of having students guess the consequences or "how far" they can go in their own misbehavior before there is a response.

Tell students how they can "earn" the right to work with a friend, to receive a grade of "A," to become a group leader. You might want to post these consequences when you post your rules. For example, you might note, "After you complete your work and it has been checked, you may begin your 'free reading' time." Too often the negative is emphasized: "When you talk the first time, your name goes on the board. The second time, you receive a check next to it, meaning that you will have additional homework that night." As the number of checks is added to the student's name, additional adults are needed to underscore the punitive nature of the response.

These responses underscore expectations. When students are told what they may do when they complete their work, the message is that the teacher expects them to complete it. But when the teacher tells them what will be done when they talk during class, they are being told that the teacher expects them to talk.

Sometimes teachers of resource or Content Mastery classes feel frustrated about their inabilty to assign grades to student work, since this is often done by the mainstream teacher. Other times, the resource teacher assigns a grade, but the student and family do not feel it is as important as grades in content area subjects. So, they note, the power of the grade as positive or negative consequence is lost.

This does not have to be the case at all. Instead of using the grade as a weapon to control students, educators should view it as a means of responding to their efforts, a benchmark for the degree of student effort and improvement. When teachers do not "officially" grade students, they actually have more flexibility in the areas to which they choose to respond.

For example, if we have a student who has refused to do any written work because of a previous history of failure, an "A" grade can be awarded for any effort. As the student begins to complete work more frequently, grades can be assigned for improvement or creativity of ideas. Or no grades have to be given at all if this task is performed by the regular classroom teacher. Positive comments can be written on paper, stating specifically what was liked (not disliked) about the effort. Then the student can be taught directly in the areas where improvement is needed. There are many teachers who would love never having to assign grades.

Teachers can differentiate the rules and assignment of grades based on student capability levels. While this initially may seem unfair, it actually demonstrates more concern about individual student behavioral and academic goals. Sean is a major problem for Barbara because he constantly is out of his seat and calls out while she or others are talking, demonstrating low impulse control. On the other hand, Mark is an angry child. He has outbursts of almost uncontrollable aggression where he attacks other children without provocation. While both students lag years behind in reading and have expressive language disorders, their behaviors cannot be handled the same way.

Rules for Sean would include staying at his desk for specified periods of time, gradually extended as he gains control. He would be allowed to move around at his desk freely as long as he is completing his work. His calling out could be modified by his completing a daily graph with Barbara, monitoring the reduction in frequency of verbal impulsivity. He could be praised and rewarded as the graph shows a decline in the objectionable behavior.

Since Mark is potentially injurious to others, Barbara would have to establish an additional set of rules for him, one that the other students might not need. She would help him indicate when he was feeling particularly angry by telling her, and later, by going to a quiet, neutral area where he could regain his composure. Any outburst that did occur would result in his being placed in a "time-out" area until Barbara felt he was ready to return to class. He would need to demonstrate no outbursts for a specified (and gradually extended) time to earn the right to work or socialize with other students. He would be praised for positive behavior during nonaggressive periods.

In designing these rules and behavioral plans, Barbara has to attend carefully to student capability levels. A child with Attention Deficit Hyperactivity Disorder such as Sean may not be able to follow an ironclad rule such as "Students must sit quietly at their desks"; he may need to stand sometimes or to move around because of his neurology. On certain days, Mark may not be capable of participating with other students at a learning center or an Academic Club. He would then work by himself until interactions were possible. "But I can't have separate rules for everyone in the class," notes Barbara, "or I'd go completely crazy." It's not necessary to have totally separate rules, but to have flexible ones for the entire group and then to add additional rules for disruptive students.

This concept of rule flexibility has to be interpreted carefully. Flexibility does not mean lack of enforcement of rules or immediate consequences. It does mean that there are realistic behavioral expectations based on observation of student capabilities. Hyperactive students cannot sit still for hours; distractible students will have problems attending to lectures. Teachers can hold students accountable for following rules realistic to their capabilities and can intensify demands for appropriate student behaviors gradually as students are more able to reach the behavioral standards of the entire group.

COOPERATIVE LEARNING

Johnson, Johnson, and Holubec (1986) and Slavin (1983) have designed one of the most exciting approaches to helping students learn to interact appropriately with others while improving their academic skills. "Cooperative Learning" is just that—a means of helping students establish joint goals and work together to achieve them. While the structure of Cooperative Learning naturally fits within the discussion of grouping arrangements in Chapter 2, it is included here to underscore how the organization of student learning can affect individual and group behaviors.

Within the structure, groups of approximately four students of heterogeneous skills are assigned by the teacher on a flexible basis, with groups rotating occasionally (approximately every one or two months). There are specified rules for individual behavior within the group, such as the requirement for each member to contribute information, ask for help, and in turn, give help as needed, and to make sure that all members of the group understand the concepts (Johnson et al., 1986).

Each group member is assigned a role, such as the "Resource Manager," who passes out and picks up group materials; the "Facilitator," who keeps the members on task, encourages their participation, and checks their understanding of material covered; or the "Recorder" who does any required writing for the group.

Teachers are to be sure that students understand the requirements of the task and their final goal and then monitor each group's efforts. Teachers are not to answer questions of individual students, but to allow the group to respond. The teacher intervenes only when the answer is unclear to the entire group.

The benefits of Cooperative Learning are clear. Students learn to work together instead of competitively, improving social skills. Students provide feedback and encouragement to each other, and as a result, motivation. This structure often is most successful for students who tend to be aggressive, acting-out, or on the contrary, apathetic, because of the group behavioral monitoring that occurs. The structure also provides a consistency lacking in some children's homes and which they usually enjoy because of its predictability.

Cooperative Learning tends to be much less effective for high achievers who can be forced to work at lower academic levels in their groups in order to include students with weaker academic skills. Many teachers select materials appropriate to the reading or overall achievement levels of the lowest academic skills so that all students can read the materials or understand the information. While this is helpful to the students at that level, the average and gifted students are not challenged and may gain little from the activity. Having students serve as group timekeepers when they are capable of exploring higher-level conceptual skills is often a waste of their time. Cooperative Learning, as with any single structure, should be used when it is appropriate for achieving instructional goals. Many teachers feel it is the only way to instruct learners because of its cooperative elements; however, teachers need to improve the academic skills of *all* students, and at times working individually or competitively may be a better means to this end.

Barbara asks, "But can I use Cooperative Learning in my resource classroom? And can it be used in Content Mastery? Is there a way to structure these groups to actually accomplish something when students are coming in and out of my room all the time?" Yes, as long as you can be flexible and modify the system to meet your needs, not try to modify your students' needs to fit the system. Cooperative Learning might provide just the preventative discipline structure you need. Guidelines might include:

1. Be sure that you use the Cooperative Learning groups as *reinforcement* for your teaching, not as a method of direct instruction. While students do learn from each other, they do not have your mastery or skill as a teacher and usually simply will provide the answer when placed in the teaching role. Additionally, students with learning differences often need specialized methods that are in our expertise area because of extensive training. A third- or twelfth-grader does not have this knowledge.

2. Break a few of the system's rules if you need to—the student is the reason teachers are in the classroom. For example, you might use the small-grouping structures discussed in Chapter 2, placing students more homogeneously in groups when appropriate. Although they may be on the same skill level, they can still learn from each other and can answer each other's questions, with everyone benefitting equally from the discussion.

3. At other times, you can keep the integrity of the method by grouping students heterogeneously, especially when following the content-based units or establishing the Academic Clubs (Smith, 1981) described in Chapter 2. The Cooperative Learning structure can be used for answering teacher-designed questions on content material students have explored individually or in pairs, allowing each member to provide information to the group and sense a contribution from their own research.

4. In rooms using Cooperative Learning, students often read aloud and discuss content in groups. Since students with learning differences usually have a broad span of reading levels, instead of having them read materials, you might have them view media or listen to tapes and recordings while in their large or small groups and then have them respond to questions at a variety of conceptual levels with their Cooperative Learning partners. In this way, the students who are better readers will not be held back by having to read materials at lower skill levels, and they will have higher-level questions to answer. In turn, students with poorer reading skills still will be able to gain content information and will be able to answer questions at their level. Everyone can contribute to the group, a primary goal of this organizational structure.

5. Similarly, since students often learn best by doing, once grouped, they may jointly explore hands-on activities such as interviewing each other for the class newsletter, recording information into a tape recorder, or writing their own story or poem. While students would keep Cooperative Learning roles such as "Facilitator," each could still participate fully in the discussion.

The teacher's role would be to monitor their progress and help them overcome "roadblocks" by offering additional innovative ideas.

The first four suggestions work well both in resource and Content Mastery rooms, while the last one more likely would be successful in resource. Since Content Mastery teachers often complain that they are functioning as tutors instead of teachers, they should take the initiative to redesign the structure of their classrooms so that they can instruct students in ways *different* from the regular classroom, not merely by having them reread the same material or by explaining it to them. For example, tapes of books they are reading can be very helpful; within the Cooperative Learning structure in a Content Mastery unit, students could listen first to the tapes of their regular classroom texts and then participate in groups to answer the questions given by their regular education teacher. Students could "coach" each other on the information so that they would be better prepared to participate in the regular classroom.

Since students may come to the Content Mastery unit from a variety of classes at any one time, a number of subject and grade levels could be included in group activities across the room. Each group could be performing relatively independently under teacher supervision. There is no reason why every student in the Content Mastery, or resource, rooms should be working on the same assignment as the same time. The very structure of the system allows for a discipline system within diversity.

SUMMARY

Chapter 3 included discussion of the types of student behaviors teachers find most difficult, ranging from aggressiveness and defiance to apathy or "goofing off." We noted that although teachers feel the effects of these behaviors, they rarely are the cause, that students often bring these behaviors with them because of outside influences or needs for attention. Therefore, it is particularly important that teachers not personalize behavioral infractions by blaming themselves or students directly, but that they concentrate on which changes are most disruptive of learning and how to effect change.

As a first step in developing an effective discipline for their classrooms, teachers were asked to consider a series of questions to help them determine their own needs and preferences, including concerns such as which behaviors they find most conducive and detrimental to learning, rules for appropriate behavior, consequences, and ways of assigning grades.

Consideration then was given to ways of grouping students for instruction that can help prevent discipline problems. Cooperative Learning was used as an example of an instructional method that contains enough structure and consistency to direct students into more intense time on-task. But even with heavily prescribed programs such as this, teachers need to be flexible, always considering student learning styles first, modifying the system to help the student. Ways of using modified Cooperative Learning in the resource and Content Mastery classrooms were included, with an emphasis on using motivational techniques, including unit study, "Academic Clubs," a variety of media, and varied grouping arrangements.

Chapter 4 includes discussion of successful discipline systems so that teachers can direct the classroom with minimal interference from student behavior problems.

Chapter 4

DISCIPLINE SYSTEMS THAT WORK

During their first year, new teachers often are given a broad array of advice from their colleagues regarding establishing a discipline system. Some say, "Never smile 'til Christmas," and others make comments such as "You'll establish your own system" or "Adapt according to your own personality," underscoring a sense that there is little logic or planning in disciplining students, that the system develops naturally, somewhat intuitively.

As Canter (1976) notes, no one would want a brain surgeon to do exploratory surgery intuitively. Are teachers any less professional when they have the job of raising future citizens and leaders? While the setting of an operating room initially appears more important in its nature, the significance of guiding scores of young people in taking control of their own behavioral patterns is also a critical task.

CLASSROOM BEHAVIOR MANAGEMENT SYSTEMS

There are a number of classroom discipline systems that work. In his excellent book, *Building Classroom Discipline*, Charles (1989) discusses a variety of models of controlling and redirecting misbehavior, based on the work of several theoreticians and practicioners. It is important to note that there is no one system that is best for every teacher or class of students, but there may be aspects within many of the systems that would allow a teacher to develop a personal discipline plan. This is very different from the "winging it" philosophy so frequently espoused in the past: teachers have a broadened knowledge base, a plan in advance, and a series of back-up measures upon which to rely. The sense of confidence this gives means that educators *can* control their classrooms and use their time and efforts to teach students.

These primary discipline systems offer a structure within which students with learning disabilities tend to perform optimally. Following are descriptions of some of the most promising so that you can select those aspects that best support the teaching-learning environment in your classroom.

Behavior Modification

While Skinner (1971) himself never devised a discipline system for the classroom, his ideas, especially in discussing reinforcement theory, have been adapted to the control of student behaviors by a number of other authors (Axelrod, 1977; Ladoucer & Armstrong, 1983; Sharpley, 1985). Behavior modification has been one of the most successful methods used with children with learning differences, likely because it relies on a base of structure and consistency, and is often motivational in its reward structure.

Including adaptations of subsequent behaviorist researchers, the "neo-Skinnerian" model emphasizes that for most individuals the reason for performing a particular action is in the consequences that action will have. If individuals feel that behaving in a specific way will result in the desired outcome, they are more motivated to behave accordingly. And each time they are reinforced for that particular behavior it becomes more deeply embedded in their daily repertoire until they no longer need constant responses—intermittant ones will do. If a behavior is not reinforced at first, it tends to become weaker, underscoring that constant reinforcement initially instills the behavior the most.

Behaviorists indicate that the best way to "extinguish" undesirable student behaviors is to not reinforce them, to ignore them. However, when an act occurs that cannot be ignored, such as physical aggression toward another student, punishment is used to change the behavior.

Aspects of behavior modification always have been used between people, and the classroom is no exception. Praising student answers to questions, assigning grades for work completed, or removing students when disruptive have been management tools teachers understand. There have been problems with implementation, however: teachers usually have not been systematic, they often have reinforced behaviors that they intended to extinguish, and they have relied on the negative instead of the positive to shape behaviors. Even in their sporadic use, teachers have relied on these techniques because they do change behavior.

Following are some guidelines that may make your behavior management system even more successful.

Select Reinforcers That Are Important to Students

Not all students respond strongly to praise or grades, especially if their needs are more basic or concrete. Yet, because certain reinforcers usually have been meaningful to teachers during their own schooling, they tend to rely on them almost totally. Teachers should find out what their students most need or enjoy and select these reinforcers.

Some students are very concrete and will perform desired work for *tangible reinforcers* such as food (raisins, popcorn) or objects (pencils, posters). Usually students with the most severe behavior problems are at this level: receiving an object is a visible sign of their success, one that they can show others and use to bolster their own self-esteem. Many times these tangible objects are received as the result of a token economy, where a student receives a token or mark each time a designated task or behavior is performed successfully. The student may "cash in" tokens for a tangible object or may accumulate them for a more significant reward at another time.

Other students enjoy *activity reinforcers*, where they can earn the right to perform a preferred activity (working with a friend, free reading) by completing a less preferred one (a spelling assignment, homework). This theory is based on "Grandma's Rule"—first you do what you are requested to do, then you get to do what you want to do. (In Grandma's house, "First you eat your peas, then you eat dessert" or "After you clean your room you may go to the movies.")

Move Students Through the Hierarchy of Behavioral Levels

Consultants in one school district advised teachers to avoid using behavior modification because "the students were becoming too dependent on receiving something every time they did their work." This advice was particularly surprising since the district had embraced this very system a few years before, to the point of insisting that their special education teachers attend workshops and cooperate within schools for broader coordination. Yet, there was consensus that the system had failed.

What had happened? Initially, the levels of behavior management and their relationship had not been understood clearly. These levels are listed in Figure 4-1. In initiating the system, most teachers had started all students at the lowest level on the behavioral hierarchy, that of tangible, especially food, reinforcers. While the teachers felt that they needed to be fair and to give to one what they were giving to another, they did not realize that many students would work well for rewards at higher levels, such as taking a message to the office or even just a smile.

As a result, many students who did not require tangible reinforcers began to depend on them, even to consider them their due. "What will I get for completing math?" became the question of many who had previously done their math without a particular reward. The teachers became concerned as they watched previously capable students regress. This problem was not uncommon during the initial stages of use of behavior modification in special education. As a matter of fact, Behaviorists frequently were called "M&M pushers."

For the system to work, it must be followed correctly. Teachers are the best judges of where students are in the behavioral hierarchy shown in Figure 4-1. If a child has extreme behavioral needs or lacks any motivation to perform a task or is economically disadvantaged, tangible rewards usually are necessary. A young girl with cerebral palsy once took her first steps for one piece of candy offered by her physical therapist. She previously had refused to try to walk because she found it painful. There was not a dry eye in the room, especially her mother's, and no one would have begrudged the girl a boxful

---

Hierarchy of Behavioral Rewards
Most Basic
1. Food, tangible rewards
2. Tokens, representing gains toward a tangible reward

Advanced, External
3. Graphic reinforcers (charts of gains, "happy faces")
4. Activity Reinforcers (messages to office, drink of water, working on class project)
5. Praise and approval from others

Note: Praise should accompany all reinforcements at prior levels

Advanced, Internal
6. Self-Praise: personal acknowledgment that we have done well, despite responses of others

---

Figure 4-1. Hierarchical levels of behavioral rewards.

of candy for her valiant efforts. Yet, within weeks, because of the praise of others and her own feelings of accomplishment, the same girl continued her faltering steps with no tangible reward at all.

Once a student begins previously refused work efforts based on a tangible reward system, the teacher should make these rewards intermittant so the efforts continue but the student does not become reliant on material reinforcers.

The next step is to begin substitution of tokens or marks for tangible rewards, encouraging students to accumulate them as long as possible. This process allows students to begin to delay gratification, a task difficult for many children with Attention Deficit Hyperactivity Disorder or children from homes where they cannot count on adult consistency. When students find that they can earn a more important reward by waiting a few days and that adults can be counted on not to forget and to give them what was promised, the "weaning" process has begun.

Teachers then can move to graphic reinforcers, where students receive a mark on a chart or a symbol (stars, stickers). While traditionally these markers have been given to younger students, a number of educators chuckled during the recent "scratch 'n sniff" sticker craze when girls at a local high school viewed the stickers as prize objects. For the first time many of them performed their work with alacrity, causing their teachers to buy stickers by the bookful. Additionally, marks on charts, similar to the tokens, can be tallied for a greater reward; the marks do not need any additional reinforcement since they can stand by themselves as positive reinforcement.

Activity reinforcers particularly are valuable in special education where students tend to have a high activity level, a short attention span, and need to move around. Any school activity the student likes can fit into this category, making the list extensive. But the teacher should pair the reward with praise and remind the student *why* the reward has been earned. ("John, I'm so proud of you for finishing all your math problems today. You've earned the right to put up the books." Or to get a drink of water, or to help Kathy with her math.)

Social reinforcers are near the top of the hierarchy since they command the most amount of self-discipline for the least tangible reward. These are the kind teachers tend to enjoy giving most. Ranging from positive words to a wink or smile, or just standing in proximity to students, they indicate that teachers care about them as people and approve of their work. While they would like to start at this higher reward level with all students, educators usually cannot. While it was often believed that only students who came from homes where their other needs were met were at the social reinforcement level, as Barbara notes, times have changed, and there is a new group of students who respond beautifully to these rewards. These are the students whose emotional needs too often are neglected and who will do anything for attention. Receiving praise or a hand on the shoulder from a teacher tells them that the most important person in the classroom feels that they too are important and helps the growth of self-esteem. For everyone, a reminder of the approval of others is important reinforcement for repeating the task at a later time.

Like adults, students do not like to give things up. Once they have been earning objects and activities as reinforcers, they are reticent to stop receiving them and to work for praise alone. This leap from more basic levels on the hierarchy often is the most difficult.

There are two ways to handle this transition. The first is to start students on the rung of the reinforcement hierarchy where they naturally belong. A student from a home where parents are "too busy" to spend much interactive time will work well for praise alone. To avoid any jealousy, as you are giving a student on a lower reinforcement level a few pieces of popcorn for completing an assignment, you casually may offer some to the student working for praise. It is surprising to find that while they may accept it at first, they often turn it down after time, indicating it is not important to them. Their sense becomes that you are not slighting them by not offering tangible rewards, but that they "don't need them."

The other way to guide students from lower reinforcement levels to social reinforcers is to include praise all along as a natural accompaniment for any task or behavior for which you approve. Then become intermittant in awarding tangible or activity reinforcers, but keep praising students constantly. They will begin to change their dependence to social reinforcement.

While most theorists stop at the social reinforcement level, personal reinforcement appears to be even higher, since it emphasizes a quality observed in the most-fulfilled individuals. Even adults tend to rely too heavily on the praise of others for a sense of self-worth. If students, parents, colleagues, and principal do not tell teachers often (and they rarely do) that they are doing a good job, teachers tend to doubt themselves.

Students at the self-praise level perform their schoolwork successfully because they enjoy success and a feeling of accomplishment. While they enjoy the praise of others, this praise is not necessary for them to do their best. It is interesting to observe a trait of perfectionism in so many students with learning disabilities. While they may punish themselves when they do not perform very well, they also feel wonderful when they achieve success. This tells educators to provide tasks on which students can be successful, allowing for their personal sense of accomplishment and adding to the positive atmosphere of the classroom. Students can begin the road to self-praise through hearing teacher comments about how well they perform tasks, specifically noting precisely what they did ("I like the neatness on that paper today" or "I'm really pleased your homework is in on time"). As teachers become intermittant with external praise, students will begin to internalize by using self-praise.

Ignore Behaviors You Want to Extinguish

Teachers need to understand that one way or another students will get attention, positive or negative, and they regard either type of attention as better than no attention at all. When Barbara yells at Mark or gives him the "evil eye" (which teachers feel cuts a student to the core), she actually is encouraging him to misbehave again. He knows that he has captured not only her attention, but that of the rest of the class. His misbehavior is being rewarded.

When he misbehaves, especially with "goofing off" behaviors (daydreaming, fooling around, not completing assigned work) or with disruptions (calling out, clowning around), Barbara should ignore what she can. At the same time she should turn to students in Mark's proximity who are behaving well and compliment them or give them an unexpected activity reinforcer ("Ellen, you've been working so hard that I'm going to let you take a break and carry this note to the office").

Attending to Ellen's good behavior sends two messages. It tells her that in this classroom, good behavior is rewarded, and it tells Mark that negative behaviors do not warrant any rewards or attention.

Time Out

"But you don't know Mark," Barbara interjects. "I can't ignore him when he's walking around the classroom disturbing others, sometimes even hitting them. He makes fun of Ellen's weight, Joe's sister, and encourages Juan to fight with him. I know he gets attention from all of us when he does these things, but I have no other way to handle him."

She is right. Teachers cannot ignore students who are physically or verbally abusive or who are ruining the learning environment for others. But the worst thing to do is to make their behavior the center of attention. The first day of school, when setting rules, the key is to explain to students which of their behaviors absolutely will not be tolerated. When they lose control, they should be sent immediately to a "time out" center where they cannot participate in or even observe what is happening in the classroom.

"Time out" can be as basic as a chair or desk set off by a natural room partition such as a bookshelf or filing cabinet, or as sophisticated as a totally separate area. Since special education teachers notoriously are given less space, the latter is usually the case. While some experts advise having a student spend a set amount of time in this isolated placement, flexibility appears to be the key to its success.

Resource teachers in Alamo Heights Independent School District, San Antonio, Texas, use the time-out rules listed in Figure 4-2. They note that students tend to behave best in time out if they know exactly what is expected of them. This structure is particularly important during an acting-out or crisis episode; the posting of these rules in the time-out area acts as a reminder.

While these are for elementary-age students, they can be adapted to secondary students, as listed in Figure 4-3. Encouraging older students to write down exactly what has occurred during the behavioral infraction gives them an opportunity to vent their feelings and allows the teacher to see the incident through their eyes. It also indicates situations that may "trigger" outbursts in this student so that in the future these situations can be avoided. At the end of the day or when the students are sufficiently calm, they meet with the teacher and discuss what happened, clarifying the issue. Ways that the student can refrain from behaving this way in the future and considerations for similar future situations also should be discussed. This use of time out thereby can help prevent future outbursts.

Punishment

While it is easier to punish than to reward, punishment should be avoided and should be used only when absolutely warranted because it detracts from the positive atmosphere of the classroom. However, when students' behaviors are extreme,

---

"Time-Out" Behaviors: Elementary Grades

1. Sit in chair quietly; teacher sets timer.
2. Keep feet on the floor; face forward.
3. Fold hands or write ABC's/Numbers.
4. Keep still while timer is on.
5. Timer rings; put name on paper(s).
6. Stand up; push in chair; you may go.

Figure 4-2. Rules for "time out"—Elementary Grades. *Source:* Mrs. Nancy Ellis, resource teacher, Alamo Heights ISD, San Antonio, Texas.

"Time-Out" Behaviors: Secondary Grades

1. Sit quietly for amount of time indicated by teacher.
2. Do not attempt to speak to anyone in the class.
3. Write down exactly what happened, step-by-step, before you were placed in time out.
4. When the teacher says you may leave, return quietly to your seat.
5. Begin your work. Talk to no one.

Figure 4-3. Rules for "time-out"—Secondary Grades.

there tends to be an acknowledgment by everyone that punishment is necessary.

Sending a student to the principal's office for misbehavior often is not perceived as a punishment but as a reward. The student gets to leave the room, often in the company of another student, to wave at or to talk with other students on the way, and usually to sit and wait, sometimes for a long time, for the principal. Often, harried secretaries employ these students to carry messages to other classrooms. The student also visits with everyone entering the office. Additionally, the principal tends to feel that the teacher is incompetent because of an inability to handle discipline problems within the classroom. No one benefits.

This situation is similar to that of the student who is "punished" by being seated outside the classroom in the hallway. Clearly not a "time out," this seat allows the student to watch everyone go by, providing a social reward. Students do not change behaviors when they believe their actions are being rewarded.

While behavior modification has been one of the most effective methods of discipline management in the classroom, it is not the only way. Other theorists have developed additional strategies. You do not have to choose one system and use it to the exclusion of others. For example, while many teachers like operant conditioning's emphasis on prescribed consequences for behaviors, they enjoy additional discussion with the student or using a variety of methods to prevent misbehavior. Following are suggestions by others that you may find helpful in establishing a discipline system.

Jacob Kounin. Kounin's (1977) research supports three important considerations for teachers in managing student behavior: the "ripple" effect, "withitness," and "overlapping." The "ripple" effect occurs when the teacher reprimands one student and at the same time influences the behavior of students witnessing the reprimand. To strengthen this effect, the teacher should state clearly what the unacceptable behavior is and why it should end. The teacher's attitude should be one of seriousness of intent without demonstrating real anger or punishment. As observing students note the teacher's ability to take charge when students are misbehaving, they tend to avoid performing the same acts that received a disciplinary response. Kounin found the ripple effect to be most successful with students in elementary grades. Responses of high school students tended to be based on the popularity of the teacher: highly regarded teachers brought about more immediate responses from the entire class.

"Withitness" describes a teacher's ability to know what is going on in all areas of the classroom at the same time. Even when teaching one group of students a new concept while others are working on individual activities, the teacher should be totally aware of what all students are doing. When students understand that the teacher does know what each of them is doing, they tend to be more on-task. Timing is very important also, since a teacher who is highly observant of student behaviors can stop a problem before it increases in intensity or spreads to other students. By being aware of students' actions, teachers can select which student initiates the problem, avoiding punishing the wrong one.

"Overlapping" stems from the teacher being able to handle more than one classroom activity at a given time. For example, if the teacher is listening to students read in a small group and another student needs to have a math or spelling paper checked for accuracy, the teacher can stay with the reading group while glancing at the paper. Or if the teacher is talking to one student about classwork and another begins to misbehave, the teacher can signal the student to desist the inappropriate behavior while continuing to listen to the original conversation. Since there are so many interruptions in our classrooms, "overlapping" is a prerequisite for effective teaching so that the teacher does not have to constantly stop activities of the entire group.

Haim Ginott. Ginott (1971) emphasizes a social-emotional approach to classroom discipline. He places concern for student feelings and self-esteem as the primary goal of the classroom. His methods are supportive of establishing the positive classroom environment discussed earlier. Ginott writes that the way teachers talk to students when correcting their behavior is critical: they should never be sarcastic or attack students' characters, but instead remind them of the correct behavior. For example, when a student is off-task and looking around the room, the teacher might comment, "It's time to finish your work," instead of "You're always daydreaming. Why can't you ever finish your work?" The latter comments reflect on the student's personality and result in hurt feelings and lowered self-esteem.

This model also relies on cooperation as a basis for student behaviors, again respecting student abilities to perform independently. The resource or Content Mastery teacher might greet students as they enter the room and briefly state, "Let's get started right away," respecting student abilities to find their folder or take out assigned activites and begin working.

When students are upset or not working well, Ginott believes that teachers should acknowledge feelings by listening supportively and by asking how they can help. This is another way that the teacher demonstrates caring and invites student cooperation. Importantly, teachers should model the behaviors they would like to see in students.

Ginott's model is best for developing positive classroom affect, for working with apathetic types of students, often getting them to work for the first time, and with students requiring attention that they may not be receiving at home or in other classes. However, it is rarely successful with more aggressive, defiant students or with whole classes that are out of control.

Lee Canter. One of the most forceful ways of dealing with difficult-to-manage students and classes has been popularized by Canter (1976). Called "Assertive Discipline," this system borrows techniques from a number of other models, especially behavior modification, with its reliance on rewards and punishments as consequences, as well as a use of Ginott's method of addressing the situation and never responding negatively to the student's character. However, Canter has provided an easy-to-implement, direct system, which has been adopted by numerous school systems in order to provide a consistent program for managing student behaviors.

Teachers tend to like Canter's system because it is forceful and allows them to "take control" of the class. They are told they have rights in the classroom, especially the right to teach, to expect appropriate behavior from students, and to receive support as needed from parents and administrators. Students similarly have rights, specifically to have teachers who do not tolerate inappropriate behaviors and to participate in a classroom where they can learn. Class members are not permitted to take away these teaching-learning rights, and if they choose to misbehave and interfere with the teaching-learning process, they have to face consequences.

From the beginning of the year, teachers should have set consequences for breaking classroom rules. Typical consequences include loss of favored privileges or activities, time-out, detention, meeting with the principal, and being sent home. Canter emphasizes that these consequences should be discussed with the principal and they should be sent home in a letter discussing classroom rules and asking the parents for their support. Teachers should select only negative consequences that are appropriate and which they can enforce; if they need to add additional incentives for certain difficult-to-manage students in the class, they can explain to other students that everyone is different and some students need extra support to change certain behaviors.

While Canter (1976) encourages teachers to alter the system based on individual needs, his basic behavior plan includes a six-step procedure. Steps range from writing the student's name and subsequent checkmarks on the blackboard to serve as warnings, next phoning parents to explain misbehaviors, then meeting with parents and the principal, and finally, suspending the student from school. Clearly, immediate, consistent response by the teacher, based on support by parents and the principal are critical in enforcing the system.

While some view Canter's program as too harsh, it can be very effective in establishing discipline for a difficult-to-manage class and works well to prevent major behavioral outbursts, such as defiance and aggression, by identifying the behavior and working to stop it before it accelerates. Some of Kounin's

(1977) ideas discussed earlier are critical here, such as "withitness," where the teacher is aware of everything going on in the room, as well as the "ripple" effect, where students observing the teacher's immediate response to student misbehavior know that the teacher "means business" and that their behavior should be changed accordingly.

A major problem in the implementation of assertive discipline is that teachers too often emphasize the negative consequences of a behavior and far less often reward the positive. Canter does note that positive consequences are critical, ranging from teacher's praise to special rewards and privileges, to positive notes home and group rewards. However, many teachers concentrate on the negative check system and downplay the positive.

The popularity of this system underscores that it does work for many teachers. Students like Sean might benefit from its structure and consistency. Yet there must be enough flexibility to respond to his Attention Deficit Hyperactivity Disorder needs, such as increased movement and impulsivity. Barbara might provide frequent rewards for on-task behaviors by allowing him to get a drink of water or bring a paper directly to her when completed, so that neurological drives over which he has less control are not objects of punishment. In this way, Sean would be required to follow all the rules of the class in the same manner as other students, but Barbara would be giving him the short breaks that he requires.

Esprit de Corps

Classes often have personalities. Some are quiet or serious; some are passive; others are overly active; some have a sense of humor; others never understand teacher puns. If teachers watch classes carefully during the first weeks, they can observe the interpersonal dynamics and predict the developing personality. However, as with individuals, the personality did not develop in isolation, but as a result of interactions—the teacher's included. Educators tend to underestimate the impact of their own teaching style and structure on the spirit of the group, on their morale and desire to behave and learn.

Charles (1989) underscores how groups develop a sense of purpose and a direction. But it is up to the teacher to direct the class so that group purpose helps to meet individual learning needs. When an entire class is out of control and the teacher no longer is able to maintain discipline, it often is because there was never a cohesive structure developed initially that provided a positive direction. Charles notes that the first step in creating a sense of togetherness is to develop the feeling that the class is a unit that spends many daily hours together and everyone can have pride in the accomplishments of the group. While teacher enthusiasm is important, the group must have a focus, some way that they feel they are special, supporting bonding.

The teacher can provide the focus by encouraging and recognizing success by individuals and the group. Charts are excellent ways to demonstrate gains. Supportive use of incentives, as suggested by Jones (1987), may be necessary at first, but when paired with teacher and group praise, they gradually can be faded because positive group identity becomes a reward in itself. Slower performers begin to receive encouragement, not just from the teacher, but from their more academically adept peers in resource or Content Mastery. Higher achievers are given strong regard by other group members, and in turn they often become more tolerant of others. *Attention* from teachers and peers is at the basis of developing a positive class personality, a strong morale.

In groups with a well-established esprit de corps, there are few discipline problems because students want positive attention and approval from other group members. A supportive class personality is based on respect for the teacher and any individual member showing disrespect is quickly ostracized by peers. At times, a teacher best disciplines by letting the group direct the behavior of its own members. It is critical for teachers to demonstrate the positive attitude discussed earlier, to guide the group toward achievement goals, and above all, to have a sense of humor when things do not go completely as planned.

SUMMARY

Chapter 4 explored several theories on discipline and noted how to apply them directly to the classroom. It was emphasized that no one discipline system works best for every teacher or class of students, but that there are aspects of a number of systems that offer a structure within which students with learning differences tend to perform extremely well. Behaviorist theory was discussed, including the different levels of reinforcements that students prefer, with emphasis on how to quickly move students from the most basic rewards such as tangibles to more personally integrated ones such as praise by self and others. The way to effectively use "time out" was noted, with specified rules so that students would understand how to behave during this period.

While punishment is never a good place to start in developing a discipline system, it must be used at times to cause more extreme behaviors to desist. Appropriate use of punishment was reviewed, with emphasis on fairness and response by the entire group. Additional concepts by other theorists were included, such as the "ripple" effect, where students witnessing a reprimand are affected; "withitness," where the teacher is aware of what is going on in all areas of the classroom at the same time; and "overlapping," allowing the teacher to handle more than one classroom activity at a time, stemming behavior problems (Kounin, 1977).

A social-emotional approach to classroom discipline was discussed (Ginott, 1971), where concern for student feelings and self-esteem are critical. Relying on cooperation between teachers and students, the teacher should set the foundation by observing what students should be doing as behaviors begin to become less desirable, but by never using sarcasm or personal criticism to shape behaviors.

Assertive Discipline (Canter, 1976) was included as a more forceful, "take charge," approach. Based on specified consequences for breaking rules, such as loss of privileges, detention, meeting with the principal, and being sent home, the system relies on support from parents and school administrators. Many teachers have responded favorably to this system because it allows for immediate follow-up before discipline infractions escalate. Teachers also are encouraged to include positive outcomes for students who follow the rules, avoiding a tendency to emphasize the negative aspects of the system.

Charles' (1989) emphasis on group purpose and direction and how teachers can help develop a cohesive structure was noted as a critical concern to establishing an esprit de corps. Once this sense of togetherness is developed by the group becoming focused on a goal such as reading improvement or success in the mainstream classroom, discipline problems diminish. Positive attention from the teacher and peers, as well as teacher enthusiasm, are important factors in the class working together.

Chapter 5 includes guidelines for setting up a classroom for students with learning differences. Discussion will include critical issues such as scheduling students and record-keeping, as well as developing goals and implementing new learning strategies.

Chapter 5

SETTING UP THE CLASSROOM

Previous chapters included a discussion of a broad variety of areas, from the creation of a positive learning environment to methods of instruction and behavioral management. Yet, if teachers do not start the year properly with students and colleagues, there is slight chance of any of these working. There are some significant issues in teaching students with learning differences, including scheduling, organizing the classroom for optimal time on task, record-keeping, and planning our lessons.

SCHEDULING

"Please start with scheduling suggestions," Barbara notes. "I've inadvertently made more enemies of other teachers and even students because they didn't want me to work with them during a time which appeared on paper to be the best for all of us." Ironically, scheduling is one of the most difficult aspects of teachers' jobs. Scheduling can "make or break" teaching results for the year since the support of students and teachers for remedial efforts will be undermined if they are unhappy with the designated time. It is important to include mainstream teachers, supportive staff, and, if possible, students, in selecting the optimal time for their work with you.

The method of scheduling individual students for supportive services clearly is dependent on the type of services the student is to receive. The "pull-out" model of a traditional resource classroom is being altered by the addition of the Content Mastery room and the Collaborative model, where the specialized teacher may work with students directly in the mainstream setting or may provide ongoing support to the regular education teacher and not work directly with the student at all. The following are some guidelines for scheduling students into each of these instructional arrangements.

The Resource Classroom

Mandell and Gold (1984) suggest the following steps in developing a daily schedule for working with students in the resource room.

1. Learn the times of daily and regularly occurring events, such as library visits, recess, art, music, and physical education. Many of these activities are the highlight of students' days and your work may be bitterly resented if you interfere with these times. It is also important not to feel that nonacademic subjects are less important to students, who tend to work off excess energy, as well as to learn social skills such as cooperation during recess and physical education. In art and music they often express their emotions creatively when they have been unable to do so in language-related activities. Missing the visit to the library may mean a lack of motivation to read for pleasure, the very reinforcement for the skills being taught. Additionally, music or physical education teachers feel as strongly about the importance of their subject area as do the reading and math teachers; to assume that these classes are more expendable would be to eliminate teacher cooperation in the future.

2. Obtain a copy of each mainstream teacher's schedule to note when academic subjects are taught to this student's class.

3. Review the student's Individualized Educational Plan (IEP) to identify which instructional areas are to be taught in the resource classroom and make note when these are scheduled in the mainstream room. Figure 5-1 is an example of an individual scheduling plan for the elementary grades.

While these plans are simple to create and merely reflect the student's daily and weekly schedule, the most important information is contained in the "Instructional Needs" column. This column too often notes "Reading" or "Arithmetic" as the

Student: Kathy Lowell   Date: Fall-Spring, 1991
General Education Teacher: Special Education Teacher:
   Mrs. Hammell   Mrs. Meyers

Daily Classes		Weekly Classes	Instructional Needs
Language Arts	8:30-9:15	9:15-10:15	*Reading*
Recess	10:15-10:30	M/W Physical Education	Word recognition and analysis skills, especially phonics and Dolch words.
Language Arts	10:30-11:15	T/F Music	
Math	11:15-12:00	Th Art	
Lunch	12:00-12:45	2:30-3:00	*Math*
Science	12:45-1:30	T Library	Computation of basic facts in subtraction and multiplication.
Recess	1:30-1:45		Selection of appropriate math process to use in solving word problems.
Social Studies	1:45-2:30		
Group Activity M/W/Th/F	2:30-3:00		*Verbal Expressive Language*
Dismissal	3:00-3:15		Expansion of descriptive words, such as adjectives and adverbs, in daily conversation.

Resource Room Schedule: Reading & Verbal
                      Expressive Language   10:30-11:15 daily
                      Math   11:15-12:00 daily

Figure 5-1. Individual Scheduling Plan.

areas of learning difficulty, but does not specify what types of skill deficiencies there are within these broad content categories, such as "Reading Comprehension" and "Problem-Solving." Because most teachers assume that this plan is meant to be general and these details can be included when instruction begins, most errors in scheduling students begin here.

It is most manageable to group and subsequently teach students with the same types of learning differences. Students who are deficient in phonics or in sight word analysis have a very different disability from those experiencing problems in understanding and recalling information they read. While both word analysis and comprehension are aspects of the reading process, they are dissimilar enough that grouping these students together for remediation and skill-building may not help either one. Since the primary concern in scheduling students is to meet their learning needs, it is important to be as attuned as possible to deficiency areas in deciding which students to group together.

4. The next step Mandell and Gold (1984) suggest is to schedule the student into the resource class during the time instruction in the area of academic difficulty is being covered in the mainstream class. Yet, teachers often have a mixed response to this suggestion. Most feel that if students' skills are so deficient that they cannot benefit from the instruction in the regular class, then they clearly are better off in a remedial setting where they can receive supportive services in that skill area. However, if students have a borderline level of disability, often caused by having missed or never having fully integrated some basic concepts, it may be best to allow them to remain in the mainstream class during instruction so that they do not get further behind. Therefore, their attendance in resource class would be at a different time than instruction in that content area in a regular class.

One of the benefits of the Content Mastery model is that it allows students to remain in the mainstream class as long as they can profit from instruction. When they need additional explanation or reinforcement for full comprehension, they go the the Content Mastery room. This model has become particularly supportive at the secondary level, where students cannot easily substitute attendance in the resource class for any other content subject than the deficiency area and are "locked into" more required subject areas. Ways of scheduling students into Content Mastery are discussed later in the text.

In addition to these suggestions, *age* and *grade level* always should be considered when scheduling students. No fifth-grade student wants to attend a class with second-grade students: it is embarrassing. Do try to schedule students in age-appropriate classes, at least within a few years of each other's chronological age.

Students with the same type of disability should be placed in a specified resource class. While no one wants to categorize students so that they are stigmatized, it is important for the teacher's effectiveness (and sanity) that students with learning problems work to overcome them. The recent trend of placing children with emotional and behavioral problems in the same resource unit as students with learning problems has lessened the teacher's ability to concentrate on needed academic areas and required an emphasis on behavioral management. Resource should never become an "easy out" for teachers who cannot control students' behaviors. Its effectiveness as an academic remediation and compensation environment has become diluted.

Barbara sounds irritated this time. "I can't disagree with what you're saying, but it's much too idealistic. It doesn't matter whose schedule I review or what parameters I try to set in scheduling students in my resource class—the other teachers take control. They tell me that they'll let me have the students with learning disabilities for a limited time, as if they're doing me a favor. They tell me when the student will come, not caring if other students in resource will be of similar age groups or learning problems. But they want me to take the students with behavioral problems all the time, even beyond the hours specified in the IEP. I feel as if I have no control over schedules at all."

Barbara's problem is one experienced by most resource teachers and a primary reason that this programming model often has functioned poorly. In Chapter 6, discussion will include ways of positively interacting with mainstream teachers, but there are some immediate ways of handling this problem. The basic premise is that mainstream teachers should be approached in a professional manner that indicates that educators will work together without any individual's needs being dominant. For example, if Barbara reviews the teacher's and student's schedule before meeting with the regular teacher and tentatively has grouped together students with similar learning needs, she will be better prepared for the discussion. Then she can suggest, "I can see Sean during first or third period each day. Which is best for you?" In this manner, Barbara has given the teacher a choice, but she also has given priority to the schedule she is trying to develop. If the response is that neither time is good, instead of allowing the teacher to select a different time that may not work at all for her, Barbara might suggest, for example, alternating the days so that she can work with Sean on Monday, Wednesday, and Friday during first period, and on Tuesday and Thursday during third period.

She should not offer to give up her planning or lunch period, or she will resent the other teacher's taking control, and her time with Sean will be counterproductive. If the other teacher says that she cannot release him during first or third period, have her offer a suggestion, seeking her input in a friendly way. If she is unable to offer a viable alternative, Barbara might suggest placing Sean in a different instructional arrangement, such as a Collaborative model or Content Mastery. Usually the teacher will not want to go through the meetings necessary with parents and district officials to change the arrangement and will be more willing to compromise. If not, and if Barbara is sure that he will be a "poor fit" in her other resource classes, another arrangement might work best for all of them. Additionally, Barbara will have made the point that she is trying to see Sean when it is the most profitable learning time for him and that she is willing to be flexible personally, but that she also has constraints. By doing this in a friendly but professional manner, the mainstream teachers may have more respect for Barbara's needs in the future.

The Collaborative Model

Although the resource model and other "pull-out" programs have been the most widely implemented, they have not been the most successful in improving student skills (Gottlieb, 1982; Reynolds & Birch, 1988; Wang & Birch, 1984). The problems Barbara noted of feeling isolated and less professionally accepted than her colleagues are typical of resource teachers, who are criticized for not "fixing" children's problems in a limited amount of time and in an environment where mainstream teachers and the students themselves are often nonsupportive of their efforts. No wonder scheduling is such a difficult problem for resource teachers when the students are publicly stigmatized each time they leave the classroom and when other educators are made to feel that they must not be competent enough to handle these students, that they must send them to the expert. At times when teachers actually are pleased to see them leave, it usually is because the students are behavior problems; most "pull-out" settings are even less functional since the outcome is to remove students from the presence of the peer role models they need the most.

When resource classes have been the most effective, it often has been due to the personality of a teacher able to consult with others, possessing expansive educational training in varied teaching techniques, combined with a building administrator supportive of special education. Unfortunately, there are too many variables in this model for it to be workable in most schools.

Ways of collaborating with other educators are discussed in Chapter 6. However, the scheduling of students into two types of collaboratve models will be reviewed here since the skills may be helpful to most teachers.

Collaborative Consultation

This model is an interactive process involving a team of teachers in general and special education, administrators, parents, and when possible, the student. It is based on people working together to select and provide the most effective programs for students with special needs, allowing for a combination of expertise and a sense of "shared ownership" in a successful outcome (Idol, West, & Lloyd, 1988). Use of this model would lessen a number of the problems Barbara mentioned because there would be ongoing collaboration after the referral meeting to determine which programming options were best, whether the student should be part of a more traditional resource program at all, and if so, when the student should be scheduled to attend. Barbara would neither be the villain who is forcing others to meet her schedule nor the victim whose own teaching needs rarely are met. The team members would work out the schedule cooperatively and would generate new solutions when problems arose.

Barbara still would be responsible for proposing a "master plan" in which students should work together in groups because of related needs, but her colleagues would be more aware of the specific problems of a variety of students merely by participating in the discussions with her. Similarly, she would benefit by hearing firsthand the types of problems the students are demonstrating in the mainstream class and at home, broadening her awareness of additional skills she might emphasize.

Collaborative consultation clearly goes beyond scheduling and its benefits will be discussed more completely in Chapter 6. However, its very core emphasizes the type of cooperation necessary for placing students in the best instructional setting during the optimal time period.

Team Teaching

Some districts, such as St. Paul, Minnesota and Iowa City, Iowa, have found that "pull-out" programs are the least desirable for their students. In an attempt to serve students with special needs in as "inclusionary" a program as possible, model units have been developed where regular and special educators work together in the same classroom and share the teaching of all students. There are no restrictions on which students either teacher may instruct, allowing for fluid grouping of students by need. A primary concern expressed earlier is obviated by this system: students are scheduled individually, by pairs, and into groups based on their developmental or remedial instructional needs. Anyone requiring more instruction in a particular area, from word attack to advanced writing skills, can work with any other student and with the teacher most qualified in that area.

The strength of the program is that teachers with general and specialized training work together to share their expertise. Figure 5-2 notes the instructional roles both types of teachers bring to a team-teaching environment.

In settings using team-teaching arrangements, teachers no longer are isolated from each other and become more innovative and excited as they "brainstorm" ideas to make their room more stimulating. The general educators often comment about how much they gain from learning specialized methods from their colleagues, experiencing success for the first time in reaching "incorrigible" students. The special educators usually are surprised at the breadth of curriculum the generalist must teach in one year and at the differentiated management needs in large-group instruction. Most important, they learn from each other.

A number of the innovative strategies discussed in Chapter 2 can be incorporated easily into the team-teaching arrangement. Learning centers can form the core for individualized instruction, with teacher supervision and programmed materials. Computers are used often for reinforcement of basic skills. All students can participate in the use of media. Guest speakers and "hands-on" projects help comprehension and retention, and use of content units and "Academic Clubs" (Smith, 1981) provide additional motivation and excitement.

Scheduling takes on a different complexion in the team-teaching room, because the primary concern is which students would benefit most from this environment. Selection should be based on questions such as consideration of the degree of Attention Deficit Hyperactivity Disorder and whether this condition is severe enough to limit the student's attention in a large-group environment. If learning or behavioral needs are extreme or would hinder the instruction of others, a more restricted setting such as resource may be optimal.

As noted earlier in discussing scheduling students into the resource program, a total profile of the class should be reviewed to assure that there is a match among members. In a team situation, teachers should meet and discuss the learning and behavioral characteristics of individual students, reviewing the appropriateness of the placement for anyone with extreme

Special Education Teacher	**Regular Education Teacher**
Knowledgeable in remedial techniques	Awareness of curriculum requirements in a variety of content areas
Resource for supportive materials and equipment	Indepth knowledge of content
Expert in developing programs individualizing instruction	Familiarity with appropriate scope and sequence of content
Aware of varied behavior management strategies	Adept in directing class discussions
Knowledge of flexible small-group arrangements	Ability to implement a variety of methods, such as peer tutoring and cooperative learning within a large-group setting
Understanding of assessment techniques	Ability to work with a variety of students within the mainstream environment
Ability to identify regular education students with potential learning problems	

Figure 5-2. Team-teaching: Shared strengths of regular and special educators. Adapted from Davis, L. C. (1989). *Collaboration and collegiality among regular and special educators: Restructuring to meet the needs of students at risk.* Unpublished manuscript, Trinity University, San Antonio, Texas.

problems. Based on the class profile, a student might be better placed in a certain group or scheduled during one time of the day instead of another.

The team-teaching model can work effectively throughout high school unless students are placed in classes containing only students with basic skills, in effect creating a totally special education environment (Waldron, 1985).

Barbara notes, "I like this. I can see where not only scheduling but programming could be dramatically improved using the collaborative models. But, for example, if I team-teach with a colleague for most of the day, what will happen to my students who can't survive in that larger group and who really need more intense specialized instruction?"

Flexibility is the key. You may want to team-teach with a regular educator part of the day, likely in the morning in elementary grades and for specified class periods in secondary, but for the rest of the day, you may want to see students with more severe disabilities in your resource room. Or you may want to develop a Content Mastery support system for part of the day in addition to working in a team situation. The student's learning needs should always determine the type of instructional arrangement and schedule. If there is more than one special education teacher in a school, each teacher should select the model inspiring the most personal confidence. The easiest combination for scheduling purposes would be for one teacher to be involved in the Collaborative model for a large part of the day, supplemented by a resource room for students with more intense needs. The other teacher could have a Content Mastery class for students requiring reteaching or reinforcement for learning.

Content Mastery

A teacher using the Content Mastery model should be doing so voluntarily, since the chances of success will be far greater when there is a personal commitment. Content Mastery teachers in Carrollton-Farmers Branch Independent School District suggest the following scheduling guidelines for the first week of school:

1. Request a copy of the class schedules of all students with learning disabilities.

2. Initiate a card file on all teachers with whom they will be working. Write the teacher's name on the card, followed by all students in the class who will be assigned to Content Mastery. Color-code the cards to distinguish among grade levels or content areas for the teacher, so that varied groups of students can easily be distinguished.

3. Start a file for each teacher, including student cards, and another file for each student, including parent contact information.

4. All books and materials in the Content Mastery Center should then be labeled by subject area, and when appropriate, by teacher assignment (for example, "Biology text: Mrs. Fuller").

5. Arrange a binder for each course you will be supporting. Within the binder, there should be a divider for each teacher instructing that course. Lesson plans, exams, and study guides provided by the regular education teachers will be filed later in the binder along with additional materials added by the Content Mastery teacher.

6. In person, you might give a typed list of the names of students eligible for the program to each involved teacher. You should then discuss the program with each teacher and answer any questions or review aspects requiring clarification.

7. An important step in the organizational and scheduling process is to hold a meeting for students who will be enrolled in Content Mastery. The program should be detailed for the students so they feel secure in operational details. It is important to be positive with students so they understand the program will support their individual needs.

8. Obtain lesson plans and any necessary books and materials from teachers. In schools where lesson plans are turned into the office weekly, you might copy these with teacher permission so that you can plan in advance.

9. Begin "highlighting" textbooks for students and recording on tape any particularly difficult chapters for students to read. Usually there is a teacher assistant in the Content Mastery unit who can continue to perform these supportive tasks as the year begins.

10. Ask teachers to tell you at the beginning of the week when they will be giving tests to any of your students so that you can prepare in advance. If the students are to take exams in your class, you might discuss with teachers the preferred testing adaptations (e.g., reading the test to the student, taping it, modifying the length or format). You might prepare a bulletin board for each teacher's assignment and exam schedule so that students can begin work immediately after entering the room.

The student's actual scheduled time in Content Mastery differs from that in the resource room, because the instruction is received in the mainstream room and the student may not attend the Center during direct instruction, group assignments, class discussion or media presentations. Either the mainstream teacher or the student may suggest that it is time to leave for the Center during the following: when the rest of the class is working independently and the student has not understood the concepts, requiring reteaching; when the student is reading silently, working on a worksheet or from a text and is having difficulties; or when preparing for a test.

Because of the flexibility of this model, the amount of time spent in the Center will vary, and the student may not need to attend each day. However, the student's IEP usually specifies the minimum amount of time to be spent in the Center weekly, requiring a record of specific dates and times to meet guidelines. While this extra paperwork is viewed as a problem by most teachers, there are ways to simplify the process. The students can note the date, time they enter and leave the Center, and the subject area they studied on a "sign-in sheet" similar to that in Figure 5-3, used by Carrollton-Farmers district. On a daily basis the teacher or assistant can add up the number of minutes to obtain the weekly total, assuring that the student is meeting the minimum number required by the IEP. If it is noted that a student has stopped attending or is spending less time than that prescribed, the Content Mastery teacher can send a note or directly contact the regular classroom teacher as a reminder. If both teachers feel that the student no longer needs as much time in Content Mastery, an Admission/Review/ Dismissal (ARD) meeting should be held to shorten or eliminate participation. The record of amount of time in attendance, combined with consideration of student progress in general education during the year, also can help the committee decide about the appropriateness of this or other special educational placements in the future.

Most centers have a teacher and assistant so that one person is always there, even during planning periods and lunches. Since it is imperative to have flexibility in meeting with regular education teachers regarding student progress, Content Mastery

Six Weeks Period 1 2 3 4 5 6

Carrollton-Farmers Branch ISD
Special Education Department
Content Mastery Center
Sign In Sheet

Name_____   Date Six Weeks Ends _____

Subject Code:

1. Reading   3. Spelling   5. Math   7. Social Studies
2. Language/English   4. Composition   6. Science   8. Health
                                                                  9. Other

Date	In	Out	Subject	Length of Visits in Minutes

Total Minutes by Subject: A. Total Time in Center in Minutes _____
1. _____ 5. _____   B. Days Center Open & Student Attended School____
2. _____ 6. _____   C. Average Daily Length of Visit_____
3. _____ 7. _____   (A/B = C)

Figure 5-3. Content Mastery Sign-In Sheet. Reprinted with permission, Carrollton-Farmers Branch ISD, Texas.

teachers often find that they can leave the Center during the less busy hours requiring only one adult and flexibly can meet the planning needs of other teachers.

Many teachers find that the Content Mastery Center must be open before and after school, as well as during school hours to meet scheduling needs and to allow students to review subjects in which they are experiencing difficulty or need support in preparing for an exam. Regular classroom teachers also tend to "drop in" more often during hours convenient for them and generally are more positive when they informally corroborate with the Content Mastery teacher.

RECORD-KEEPING

But one of the greatest problems all educators face is developing the balance between teaching-learning time with students; working with other personnel; performing administrative tasks required by the school, district, and state; communicating with parents; and developing an organized system to handle the needs of all these groups. One of the greatest arenas of frustration for educators today is paperwork. A teacher needs a system of organization that allows for accurate record-keeping on a daily and composite basis.

Since there are so many ongoing demands, it is easy to rely on a "crisis management" system, where the paper needed the most urgently is the one most actively sought. Many times students are off-task, getting into behavioral difficulties while the teacher is looking for a misplaced student paper or materials necessary for the assignment. Teachers often respond with a feeling of being overwhelmed and unable to cope with these extensive demands, a developmental "burn-out."

Educators need to take control of the extensive record-keeping demands placed on them. They can start by analyzing the different types of organizational needs they have and then developing a basic system to handle each one. The types of record-keeping fall into several categories. The most demanding on a daily basis are in-class, where depending on the type of instructional arrangement, from resource to collaborative to Content Mastery, students are made aware of what they need to do, their progress, and their behaviors. Directions for activities as well as materials location play an important part in organization, so that students can begin tasks independently and not interrupt the teacher's time with other students.

The second category is the least personal, and therefore often the most bothersome to educators. It includes administrative requirements, ranging from the principal's unpopular format for writing lesson plans to state and federal regulations for tallying numbers of students served by handicapping condition. Teachers of the learning disabled often are unhappy that they not only have to meet the individual school mandates but also those of the district Special Education Department, including reams of paperwork for the ARD process and monitoring the student's IEP. Forms seem only to generate more forms and to distract educators from the job they want most to do—teaching.

Another category varies most substantially with the type of instructional arrangement, but seems to be more in-line with actual teaching responsibilities: communicating with mainstream teachers and other supportive staff. The healthiest goal of special education is to have full participation of students in general education, as active members, able to "keep up" and learn both independently and as part of the group. Teachers need to interact fully with mainstream educators if they are to fulfill this goal, and this interaction process requires record-keeping on each student. Especially in collaborative and Content Mastery arrangements, records maintained by the specialist underscore the success or failure of support systems and are the basis for program modification and change. Similarly, there must be a system for accurately tracking student success in mainstream classes, ways of documenting behaviors requiring more intense work and content areas requiring additional remediation before the student experiences failure.

Additionally, the most successful of classrooms are those where the parents are informed of their child's successes and problem areas, but where they also participate, for example, by monitoring assignments, underscoring school attendance, and verbally supporting the actions of the teacher. Accurate record-keeping, along with a system of notifying parents about their child's work, are critical to positive parent involvement.

In Chapter 6, guidelines are presented for developing cooperative arrangements with colleagues and parents, including the organizational processes necessary for having accurate information on student progress. The following discussion includes how teachers can develop a record-keeping system that reduces paperwork, but meets the needs of the first two groups: students and administrators.

Students

If teachers of special needs students were to work with only one group of students daily, demands would be far simpler. But many teachers have to keep extensive records on a number of groups in a variety of instructional arrangements, presenting an overwhelming organizational and logistical task.

"You're so right," Barbara notes. "Sometimes I forget why I'm in the classroom. I'll finally have a good day with the kids, feeling that I've accomplished something, and then the principal will be on my case because I didn't use the standard form in writing up my lesson plans. Or, with so many students in the room daily, I can't find the file that I need for reinforcement materials for one or two children. When this happens, they become bored waiting for me and start to get into trouble. Yet my room is so small that it's really difficult for me to find space for everything. I haven't found a system that works for me and I'm feeling very disorganized."

Barbara has touched on some key issues here. Most teachers of students with learning differences have space problems because they are given the smallest of classrooms, at times rarely the size of a closet. While the administrative rationale may be that there are fewer students, requiring less space, there is little realization that these teachers often need *more* space because of the unique learning needs of their students which mandate varied grouping arrangements, space for learning centers, more materials, and additional record-keeping and storage areas. But space is expensive and these allottment policies will not change easily.

Barbara also mentioned that she feels disorganized. This issue may be the most critical since students sense how teachers feel and respond to them and the teaching-learning environment accordingly. As Smith (1981) notes, students with learning disabilities often suffer a large degree of cognitive confusion which is externally evidenced by lack of organization, such as losing assignments, messy desks and lockers, and barely being able to find their shoes in the morning. Additionally, their thought processes are distracted by environmental stimuli with the overall effect being extreme difficulty in organizing themselves to complete a task.

Since students rarely are capable of overcoming this internal and external confusion on their own, it is up to the adults in their lives to model and teach organization so that students gain these skills. Educators often have been upset by a student's life at home, noting the need for structure within the family. Yet, the classroom is the larger family, and the student who is part of an organized, caring structure for 6 hours a day certainly will begin to learn some of the same behaviors. As the classroom becomes organized, so will the students.

Barbara also mentioned her need for a system. This issue was a critical part of Chapter 4, where students learned to follow the teacher's behavioral system. Yet, it is so easy to ignore an equally important system: the development of a structured environment where students can take charge of their own time on task in an organized, efficient manner. The teacher provides the structure and oversees the consistency with which it is implemented; students understand what subjects they are to be studying, where they are to be in the room, and with whom they are to be working. The productivity and psychological comfort level of teachers and students is greater within an organized structure. But the structure must be simple, easily understood by students, and require little paperwork and planning time.

Recording Daily Assignments

The system begins the moment the students enter the room. As previously discussed, students have the greatest number of behavioral problems during transitions. Traditionally, students "clown around" as they enter the room, walk slowly to their seats, and wait for the teacher to call for their attention in an increasingly louder voice. Then the teacher takes attendance, makes a few comments to individual students, and begins directing the group, large or small, in what they need to do to get ready for the day's lesson. This "start-up" time can take 10 minutes or more of teaching-learning time, provides an opportunity for additional behavioral problems, and is unnecessarily wasted.

There needs to be a philosophical shift that gives control of learning to the students. Instead of the teacher being the source of information about where students are to be and which assignments they are to complete, students should locate this information themselves. Good record-keeping forms the basis for student independence.

In the resource class as well as in the team-teaching model in the regular class, every student should have a folder indicating all written assignments to be completed in class for the week. The more basic the form, the clearer its intent. While there are many published forms, the teacher-created ones often are best because they meet individual needs. Figure 5-4 provides an example. In the left-hand column, the teacher can list all the subject areas that are normally included in IEPs, eliminating the need to create a separate sheet for each student. There should be enough space in the blocks for teachers or students to write daily assignments.

While students will not be spending all of their class time just completing paperwork, having the week's written assignments in front of them serves two purposes: It allows them to know what is expected of them, and it provides specific work they should begin immediately after entering the classroom. Students should be instructed to go to their file and take out their weekly written assignment sheet, get the materials necessary to complete the work on the sheet, and begin that day's work. The previously wasted first 10 minutes of class can be turned into on-task time.

Depending on the discipline structure you adopted in Chapter 4, you may want to include the agreement on the bottom of Figure 5-4. With a "responsibility contract," the student is agreeing to complete the listed assignments by Friday to earn a reward or activity deemed important. The process of having the signature of the student and teacher, and at times, the principal, adds impact to the importance of the activity. While at times daily incentives may be necessary for specific behavioral changes, this weekly contract works because the student usually can complete the work by the end of the week even if there has been a difficult day or two during the week. If the reward is important enough, students may even begin coming to the room before or after school or during lunch to complete the work.

"But when can I complete all these assignment sheets?" Barbara asks. "My plate is already overflowing." Barbara is right. Teachers do not have the time to do any additional paperwork. Students should complete their own sheets under the guidance of the teacher. This goal-setting for the week's assignments allows them to take more responsibility for their own learning and to develop a sense of commitment since they have participated in the preparation of the task. For example, at the beginning of class each Monday the teacher might instruct students to take out their texts and workbooks and to tentatively write down the number of pages they can complete

In-Class Assignment Sheet

Student Name _____ Week_____

	Mon.	Tue.	Wed.	Thur.	Fri.
Reading					
Spelling					
Written Expression					
Math					
Science					
Social Studies					
Other					

Responsibility Contract: I agree to complete all of the above

work by Friday. I will then earn _____
                        (Write in selected reinforcement)

                    Student's Signature _____

                    Teacher's Signature _____

(Optional)
                    Principal's Signature _____

Figure 5-4. In-Class Assignment Sheet.

each day of the upcoming week. While a concern might be that students will become lazy and fill in fewer pages to avoid work, the opposite is true. They usually overestimate their capabilities and rate and may be unrealistic in their personal expectations. (This is the type of problem we like to have in Education.) The teacher guides the students through the planning by visiting each desk and reviewing what the student is projecting, suggesting changes where necessary. This self-planning by students works best when started a few weeks into the school year so that teachers know the levels, rate and learning styles of students, thereby being better able to guide them.

Group Assignments

Students like this system enough that they often try to impress the teacher, and themselves, about their productivity. However, teachers should be sure that individual paperwork, regardless of how popular, should be balanced by work in groups, learning centers, and unit activities. If the students are to go immediately to a group or center activity after they enter the room instead of beginning work on their assignment sheet, these directions can be posted on a wall chart where they enter the room, or color- or picture-coded for nonreaders. Instead of teachers creating new charts, another time-consuming task, a pocket chart can be used. The center or group activity can be noted or pictured on the row along the top of the chart, with students' names on separate manila strips inserted under the activity. Teachers easily can change grouping and center arrangements by moving student names as appropriate. After the first few weeks of school, when teachers have a strong sense of student achievement levels, they can follow the flexible grouping and activity patterns discussed earlier. From the beginning of the use of the charts, students should be instructed that as they enter the room they first should check the chart for their name and group. If the teacher wants students to begin their written assignments immediately instead of participating in groups or centers, the pocket chart category "Written Work" will have "All Students" posted in the pocket beneath it.

Monitoring Student Behaviors

Some students will adapt more easily to this routine than will others, especially those with behavioral problems. An important record for teachers to maintain in students' files is the behavioral progress made in following class procedures and rules, and in attending to tasks. Again, students should be in charge of recording their own behaviors, reinforcing appropriateness and making them more aware of areas in which they need to progress. While the temptation may be to develop a single sheet with class rules and to check off each student's success in following them, an individualized program will be far more meaningful.

Figure 5-5 is an adaptation of a form successfully used by teachers in Alamo Heights District, San Antonio, Texas. The form is best completed *only for those students requiring behavioral monitoring,* a factor limiting the amount of paperwork involved. Students again take charge by discussing periodically with teachers those behaviors that are interfering with learning. In the left-hand column, they write in a list of behaviors that may vary from class rules students have not been following to individual behaviors needing correction.

Based on student needs in resource, Content Mastery, and in the mainstream, the form can be completed on a daily basis for each of the classes the student attends, both in special and general education. This method is preferable because it allows for the development of a consistent behavioral plan across disciplines, encouraging all of the student's teachers to work together in changing inappropriate behaviors. Changes occur more quickly when they are reinforced throughout the school day. The student carries the form and completes it at the end of each class with the teacher by checking how successfully each behavior occurred. The discussion of categories on the form as well as teacher praise for on-task efforts are strong reinforcers.

Daily or cumulative results from this form can be sent home to parents as well as used as a basis for further collaborative efforts among educators, both in informal meetings and more formal ARD sessions. As students' behaviors improve in the designated categories, they should be omitted from the form and additional behaviors added.

At times, mainstream teachers may feel that they do not want to complete this form, or the student's organizational skills may need developing before the day-long behavioral monitoring system is implemented. In these instances, resource or Content Mastery teachers still can use the form with individual students in their own classes. While not as broadly effective, the top column in Figure 5-5 can be completed for days of the week and students can discuss their behavior with the teacher before they leave the class each day, checking the chart. At the end of the week, teachers can review progress in behavioral change or can discuss what the student needs to do to improve on-task

Behavioral Plan

Student _____   Date _____

Teachers _____   Grade _____

_____

I Will:	Language Arts	Math	Science	Social Studies
(For Example) Begin my work immediately				
Speak to the teacher politely and without sarcasm				
Stay on task, avoiding all distractions from my work				
Ask for help if my work becomes too difficult				
Participate in group work without making negative comments to other students				

Parent's Signature _____

Figure 5-5. Behavioral Plan.

work. These weekly charts can be shared with parents, giving them ideas of what to emphasize at home.

Homework Assignment Sheets

Homework is one of the best ways to provide reinforcement for material learned at school. Yet its domain primarily has become that of regular education, since special educators frequently complain that even if they do assign homework, students never complete it. "Absolutely," Barbara notes. "I've even received letters from parents saying that they don't have time to worry when their child doesn't bring books home or can't manage to bring the assignment back to school the next day. Most feel their children have enough problems with homework in academic classes and that the student should be able to get enough information in our class without my needing to send work home."

So true. Homework is often a frustrating experience for students with learning disabilities, their parents and teachers. As part of the disorganization pattern which so often accompanies the disability, students arrive home having forgotten the assignment to be completed and the books or materials necessary. While few teachers of special needs students would send home assignments that are too difficult for the student to complete independently, this situation is a problem common to general education. Parents are "burned out" at the thought of hours at the table, children angry or in tears, and total disruption of another evening, experiences to which they have become accustomed.

Yet, when students with learning disabilities carry their books on the school bus, moan along with brothers and sisters about "all the homework I have," there is a sense of normalcy, of pride in the fact that they can be expected to complete work just like other students. Steven, a middle school student with learning differences, is a good example. His mainstream teacher worked caringly with his resource teacher to give work at his level with supportive homework assignments. Yet Steven "never remembered" to take his book home and gradually became more adamant in his homework refusal. He simply would not do it. The teachers could not understand the situation since he willingly performed all his class assignments. Then his general education teacher began to note that the only book Steven took home each night was his literature text—surprisingly, since he was in resource for reading support and although it had initially been given to him, his homework assignments were never from this book, but from another more basic text issued through resource. She realized that he had such a need to be accepted by peers that he daily carried a book he could not even read instead of having his friends see him with the "dummy text." When the teachers began to give Steven his homework on printed copies of assignments or separate sheets so that he did not have to carry the book, he completed his assignments with care each night.

Beyond the academic reinforcement provided, homework is an excellent way to teach the very organizational and responsibility skills students with learning differences need. Structuring homework, like structuring the classroom, can give students direction and security and allow the family to avoid much of the usual homework trauma. The first step in supporting this structure is to only give students assignments that they can complete independently and successfully. When students know in advance that they can do the work, their initial attitude will be more positive and they usually will try. Parents also will be more supportive if they feel they do not have to assist the student constantly each evening.

The second step in structuring homework is to write the assignment on the board and explain it, or even better, to give students directions on a sheet to take home with them. So often an assignment which students feel they understand completely is not understood at all that evening.

The third step is the most critical: students need to keep an orderly record of their homework assignments which they carry to all classes, look over before leaving school, and rely on that evening to be sure all work is completed. While systems for recording assignments vary, as always, basic is best. Since too many sheets just give students more to lose, one sheet for the week is usually optimal, and it should be part of the student's notebook binder which is carried to all classes and home, so it does not get lost.

A basic form would include all subject areas listed on the side column, with days of the week listed on top. The student should be responsible for entering all assignments each class period, including upcoming exams. Since most students usually tend to be late, running from one class period to another, some teacher supervision may be necessary. The teacher giving the assignment should be sure that the student has recorded it correctly, both on the assignment sheet and when having copied material from the board or a text. So many students practice writing words they have originally misspelled, or memorize math facts they have miscalculated.

In many schools, before leaving the building at the end of the day, students with learning disabilities are required to bring assignment sheets and books or materials necessary for homework to the resource or Content Mastery teacher. While rarely taking more than a few minutes, this meeting allows the student a structure in which to learn how to prepare for homework completion. There might be a place for the teacher's signature on the homework assignment sheet to indicate that the student has met with the teacher. While it should never be necessary for parents to sit constantly with their child during homework time, it is usually good to give them some responsibility for structuring the homework area and time each evening. Suggestions for how to do this could be included in a class newsletter to parents early in the year as well as during conversations. Having parents sign the assignment sheet each night also gives them a sense of involvement in their child's work. As students become older and more responsible in completing their assignments, they can be weaned from this system, first omitting the parent's signature, and then the "check-out" visit with the teacher. However, they always should be expected to keep an assignment sheet as part of their own organization.

Administrative Records

To most special educators, the amount of paperwork required in each step of the Admission, Review, and Dismissal process is overwhelming. Understandably, they tend to resent being taken away from direct time with students to fill out forms they view as meaningless. While the forms may fulfill legal requirements, there is a justifiable sense that they rarely are useful to anyone involved in teaching. Often, records are locked in a file in the Counselor's office and not read until the hour before the next placement meeting.

While there has been a hurtful tendency for federal and state agencies to require categorization of students by area of handicap and substantiation through additional documentation of numbers of students served, in an age of public outcry over spending, "accountability" appears to be a key word. Funding always will require some paperwork and finding a method to manage it is basic to staying positive about teaching students with special needs.

The way to begin handling administrative record-keeping each year is to know what to expect. If you are new in a teaching situation or school, or if state or district rules have changed, ask both your Special Education Supervisor and building principal which records are your responsibility, when they are due, and how to obtain the specific forms to be completed. Since you are working with students in two educational settings, regular and special, you need to be aware of requirements in both areas. Being fully aware in advance will allow you to anticipate what is due and schedule your time so that you are not "under the gun" at the last minute.

This latter issue of pressure also can be lessened by keeping up with data collection on a daily or weekly basis so that final compilation of records just requires a tallying of information that you already have on file. An example of this practice was depicted in Figure 5-3, where teachers or teacher assistants daily computed the number of minutes each student was spending in Content Mastery so that they could forewarn general classroom teachers before the end of the week if students were not meeting the minimum amount of time specified on the IEP. This tallying also provides an end-of-year statement about the needs for additional or less time in the program. But with the data collected all along, there are fewer last minute demands on the teacher before the committee meeting.

Another suggestion is to involve teaching assistants, when available, in the recording of data. While collection of any information important for legal purposes must be supervised carefully and reviewed for accuracy, there are clerical tasks that a classroom assistant or office aide could do quite easily, such as attendance records, summarizing grades for students in their general education classes, creation of a filing system for administrative data, and listing of materials and equipment. Teachers must learn to delegate responsibility; as students must become responsible for their assignments both in and out of class, so assistants in the building can become more responsible for administrative record-keeping.

The collaborative model is the most supportive of delegation and shared efforts. Once a team has been established to coordinate students' programs, each member can select a record-keeping area as his or her responsibility. Many times teachers find it easier to maintain a few categories of record-keeping, such as grade checks or failure data, on all their students than to divide students into smaller groups and to maintain all records. The way the work is divided is actually the least important part of delegation. The process of teachers working together sharing information on students allows them also to share ways to overcome learning problems. In Chapter 6, additional ways to collaborate with teachers and parents are discussed.

SUMMARY

This chapter included suggestions for organizing the classroom through development of a management system. The underlying premise was that while paperwork always will be part of teaching, educators can minimize its interference with the teaching-learning process by delegating tasks to students and teaching assistants, and sharing data collection with colleagues.

Ideas for scheduling students were considered first since this area has posed significant problems for educators. It was underscored that the method of scheduling individual students for supportive services such as academic remediation is dependent on the model of service provision. Clearly the most difficult type of instructional arrangement to schedule is the traditional resource unit, since students may miss necessary information in the general education classroom when they leave and there may not be an alternate time for instruction that meets teachers' needs.

A series of steps were listed to help develop a daily schedule for working with students when the resource room is the preferred model. The steps included areas such as becoming aware of the daily and regularly occurring events in each student's day, varying from regularly scheduled classes to visits to the library; reviewing IEPs carefully so that students can be combined for instruction in resource based on the nature of their disability; offering times to the mainstream teacher that are optimal for instruction, and while remaining as flexible as possible, not placing a student inappropriately because of the demands of another teacher.

Subsequent discussion noted that despite the popularity of the resource model and other "pull-out" programs, they have not been very successful in improving student skills or in under-scoring interactions among teachers. The collaborative models of in-depth consultation and team-teaching involving both regular and special educators give faculty a "shared ownership" sense, which leans away from teacher isolation and puts students at the core of instruction. It was suggested that in collaborative situations, special educators bring knowledge in areas such as individualized instruction, remedial techniques, and alternative materials, while general educators share curricular awareness, abilities in large-group instruction, and content breadth.

Besides making scheduling easier than in resource classes, teachers have the opportunity to incorporate a variety of teaching methods, such as use of learning centers, computers, and projects involving experiential learning. Teachers schedule students within the larger class framework based on similarities in academic and behavioral needs.

Scheduling in Content Mastery was discussed next, with a series of guidelines provided to start the program off success-fully. A critical need is to create a file for each mainstream teacher sending students to the room, including lesson plans, student schedules, and specific content areas being studied. Followed by books and materials collection and including study guides and exams as the year progresses, the teacher will be able to provide excellent supportive instruction in a variety of areas.

Along with scheduling, an efficient system of record-keeping was presented as extremely important to prevent teacher "burn-out" from the weight of paperwork. On a daily basis, the records with the most impact are those systematizing work so that the student is able to begin assignments independently, to change tasks without behavioral problems so common to transitions, and to monitor gains in performance. The system is facilitated by students and teachers setting work goals at the beginning of each week and students understanding what they are to accomplish through assignment sheets they personally have completed and wall charts designed for flexible grouping. Additionally, students can have forms specifically listing the behaviors they need to change, optimally for response by special and general education teachers throughout the day.

Ways of structuring homework were discussed next, with suggestions basic to successful homework completion: giving students assignments they can perform independently and successfully; writing down the assignments so students have complete directions at home; requiring students to keep an orderly record of their assignments which they can review with a specified teacher before leaving the school, assuring that they have all materials they need.

Administrative record-keeping often was viewed as being the most unpleasant for teachers because, after taking numerous hours of time, they may not see any personal results from this information which would improve the teaching-learning process. Suggestions to make the process easier include becoming aware from the beginning of the year of the data collection and record-keeping requirements of federal and state agencies, the school, and the Special Education department, so that you can gather information on a continuous basis instead of being overwhelmed at one time. It also was noted that delegation is very important: unless the information is for legal purposes, teaching assistants and office workers can be included in compilation. In collaborative settings, individual teachers from each team can select those types of administrative record-keeping tasks they find easiest to complete, thereby sharing the work to prevent "paper burn-out" on the part of any individual.

Chapter 6 further discusses collaboration by listing a series of guidelines for effective interactions with colleagues and parents.

Chapter 6

WORKING WITH TEACHERS, OTHER PROFESSIONALS, AND PARENTS

The learning disabilities specialist must work as a member of a team. The traditional expectation of the specialist being able to work miracles with a difficult student with whom others have had little success has proven unrealistic. As Barbara has noted, the incredible problems students bring to school have become so overwhelming in their implications that no one "Super-teacher" can handle them alone. The collaborative model of instruction is becoming the strong preference in schools today, whether through consultation, ongoing collaboration, or team-teaching.

WORKING WITH TEACHERS AND OTHER PROFESSIONALS

However, despite cooperative efforts, often there is animosity between regular and special educators. The specialists may be resented because they teach fewer students, appear to have a more flexible schedule, and have additional materials, or at times, even a higher salary. On the other hand, special education teachers tend to view mainstream teachers as unknowledgeable, unskilled, and often, uncaring (Laurie, Buchwach, Silverman, & Zigmond, 1978). These perceptions pose strong blocks to cooperative planning for students.

To have teachers work together, there must be a philosophical shift from isolation to integration. Reynolds and Birch (1988) discuss the need for prevailing practices to change to preferred practices so that the student who learns differently becomes the full-time concern of specialists and generalists. They note that some of the most detrimental prevailing practices have included teachers' handling of problems alone, both in the mainstream and special class; the difficulty teachers and supervisors experience in working together as equals when discussing students, based on one professional giving advice to another; the lack of training of teachers in communication and consultation; and provision of direct services without the involvement of all the pupil's teachers.

Their preferred practices include teachers working in teams, using consultants as necessary; training in consultation techniques, allowing staff members to share and treat each other as equals; increased inservice and consultation in specialized teaching techniques so that teachers can serve all students; and efficient staff conferences directed toward problem-solving (Reynolds & Birch, 1988).

"But how do we initiate these preferred practices?" Barbara asks. "In our school, if you're the special education teacher, you've been foolish enough to want to work with tough kids and nobody has too much sympathy. As a matter of fact, I experience less animosity when I take the students from their regular classrooms than when I try to work with their teachers to implement changes in the mainstream." Without a doubt general educators often would like the problem to disappear. It is natural to feel threatened by difficult students and to want someone else to deal with them. As a result, it becomes the role of the specialist to initiate the cooperative process and to be there for support so that mainstream teachers do not feel overwhelmed.

Mainstream Assistance Teams

The best time to consult with a teacher is before the student's problems are serious enough to require special education placement. "Prereferral intervention" (Fuchs & Fuchs, 1989) refers to changes made in the student's general education classroom when developing problems are first indicated. If instructional or management changes are successful, the student often does not require formal assessment or placement in special education and can be accommodated in the less restrictive environment of the mainstream classroom.

To design appropriate prereferral intervention, Doug and Lynn Fuchs at Peabody College have developed the "Mainstream Assistance Team," a behavioral consultation model. While their program had the benefit of research staff working as consultants for school personnel, they developed a series of intervention steps that hold promise for a variety of settings. The key to their success has been in the use of a cooperative problem-solving process within teams of special and regular educators.

Perhaps one of their most interesting findings was also the most unanticipated. During the first year of their work in Nashville-Davidson County Metro Public Schools, when consultants used a collaborative problem-solving model with teachers, and the chosen interventions were determined mutually by team members, the results were not very effective. Results improved dramatically when specialists used a *prescriptive* model where they selected intervention strategies which research had demonstrated to be most successful, shared them with mainstream teachers, and provided a plan and materials to support implementation.

This finding has important implications for teachers of students with learning disabilities. When you are part of a team of teachers supporting students in regular education, you can and should provide intervention strategies to prevent failure. Your role on the team is to be the learning specialist. Problems rarely develop because mainstream teachers do not want someone with knowledge, but they often develop because the process for converting this information into a plan is faulty.

In the use of Mainstream Assistance Teams, the specialist asks the teachers to specify behavioral problems in their most difficult student. The specialist observes the student and records the behavioral problems observed, subsequently meeting again with the mainstream teacher to discuss the observation, set goals for change, and design interventions. Part of the plan often includes developing teacher-student contracts, selecting reinforcements, and fully discussing the plan with the student.

As discussed in Chapter 5, the student record-keeping system is self-monitored and recorded, putting the student at the center of the process. The mainstream teacher observes the student's progress in reaching the goal, meets with the specialist and plans modifications if necessary or develops additional goals (Fuchs et al, 1990).

The Consulting Teacher Model

While Mainstream Assistance Teams have been effective, their success is based on strong consulting skills on the part of the specialist, especially when learning problems are present, since the results may not be as immediate as with behavioral problems. Unfortunately, teachers of learning disabled students rarely are included in prereferral conferences since their work traditionally has been legislated to students already referred for services. Yet, this is where they often could be the most effective, since students' problems are more severe and difficult to overcome by the time the referral has occurred. Whether working with mainstream teachers before or after referral, the goal has to be to have them recognize that they control the learning environment and can re-structure it to prevent student failure.

One of the most important roles of the resource or Content Mastery teacher is that of a consultant with teachers in general education. In their work in the Pittsburgh Public Schools, Laurie and colleagues (1978) listed a series of steps for assisting students with learning disabilities to "make it" in the regular classroom. In some ways, these steps are a predecessor to the Mainstream Assistance Teams, although they allow for a less formalized structure and do not require as much time on the part of teachers. But they are based on a prescriptive consultancy model which has been found to be highly effective in a number of schools.

They include three prerequisites for effecting change in the mainstream: support by building administrators; time in educators' schedules to allow for planning, preparation, and meetings; and regular and special educators being able to work cooperatively. To achieve the cooperative structure, they recommend the following steps in conducting a conference with the regular education teacher.

Step 1: Determine the mainstream teacher's requirements for success. Questions to be asked might include: How is the classroom organized? How do students know what to do next? Are rules and grading practices clear? Is content presented by lecture, reading, discussion, or hands-on activities? Is the same presentation method used for everyone? How are students grouped? What materials are used and what is their level of difficulty? What kinds of tests are given?

While Laurie and colleagues (1978) feel that much is gained by having the mainstream teacher answer these questions for the learning specialist to clarify classroom demands, Fuchs and Fuchs (1989) prefer to have the specialist gather this information through personal observation in the mainstream classroom. Observation data include information such as whether there is an area for small-group work, the presence of computers, level of movement tolerated by regular education teachers, use of lecture, attention to lower-achieving students, and amount of praise for student effort. While the questions are important, this process may tend to separate the educators by having the specialist seem to be judging instead of just gathering information. Yet, even if the information is collected during a conference with the mainstream educator, the specialist should be careful not to appear formal or judgmental, attitudes that would alienate the other teacher.

Step 2. Specify which class requirements are not being met. Once requirements for success have been identified, the mainstream teacher should discuss where the breakdown is in teaching individual students with learning disabilities. Are they able to read the book? To complete the work in time? Are the students disruptive during group activities? Are their test-taking needs different? These questions by the consulting teacher may prompt the mainstream teacher to identify the focus of the problem for the first time.

Step 3. Identify the behavioral and academic skills students would need to meet mainstream class requirements. Specialists often tend to rely too much on formalized tests, the results of which often are not easily translatable into follow-up teaching in mainstream classrooms. During your conference with the teacher, ask why students are not performing well. In a secondary school setting, students often do not possess strong basic reading or computational skills and become behavioral problems because they cannot do the work. If this is the problem, the specialist should explore with the teacher the *specific areas* in which students are demonstrating deficiencies. Are basic word analysis skills intact, but comprehension skills weak in analyzing content? Are there gaps in basic math, such as the ability to compute fractions, decimals, and percentages that occurs so often in students with learning differences? Are the problems a result of Attention Deficit Hyperactivity Disorder, causing inattention, distractibility, and impulsivity?

Step 4: Brainstorm possible classroom modifications. This step is the most difficult to perform diplomatically. The consulting teacher is a specialist, most often knows the modifications that would be most successful, and, as Fuchs and colleagues (1990) note, will provide the greatest support by suggesting workable methods. Yet, the mainstream teacher needs to have a commitment to the changes, most often gained by participating in the design of the plan. The best sequence within this step is to start off with true "brainstorming," based on a sympathetic attitude of the specialist toward the need of the mainstream teacher.

The sympathetic attitude should not be feigned. It really helps if you have taught in a mainstream class, observing how a few difficult-to-manage students can ruin even the best teaching plan. A highly successful resource teacher noted, "Things go best during my conferences with teachers when I try to put myself in their place. Would I be able to handle this student in a class of 32 instead of 12? Are hostility or anger so evident that I feel relieved when the student leaves so I can regain the positive atmosphere I prefer? Would I want to have to teach this student all day instead of just for an hour? Once I finish this self-talk, I honestly can empathize with the mainstream teacher about how difficult the student is, and the teacher most often responds with appreciation that I understand what they face daily. By then, the teacher is so much more willing to try the modifications I suggest."

Be realistic in your suggestions. You must consider that the teacher likely cannot spend a lot of one-on-one time with this student and will not be able to prepare a separate set of assignments daily. You must consider class and room size, availability of materials, and content requirements of the curriculum.

If only these first steps could take place before the student initially is placed in special education, the instructional arrangements selected would be so much more successful. If members of the placement team would listen to the mainstream teacher describe classroom requirements and the student's ability to be successful, alternate arrangements such as Content Mastery or team-teaching might be implemented much sooner, before the teacher and student experience much frustration and failure. However, if this conference is occurring because the student already has experienced problems, an important option must be to consider a different setting, even if the placement committee and parents must reconvene.

Steps 5 to 7: Plan implementation. Laurie and colleagues (1978) next list several closely related steps to create change in the regular classroom. As noted previously, the action plan must be realistic for the teacher's needs; however, if the teacher continually rejects workable options, the consultant should listen to complaints empathically and then suggest modifications that might be implemented easily and show some immediate change in the student. Once teachers experience even small successes with students who learn differently, they are more willing to try more in-depth strategies.

The consulting teacher should now be available to assist the mainstream teacher in the preparation of new materials or in locating existing supportive ones. If the plan requires a change to a new teaching method, the specialist should plan time to instruct the teacher and be available for ongoing pedagogical support. When mainstream teachers are shown new methods or are given new materials, they tend to use them with groups of students, not just those diagnosed as having learning problems. In this way, many students benefit from the consulting teacher's sharing of expertise.

Step 8. Evaluate the effectiveness of the plan. If specialists feel that their job is done once they have worked out an action plan with the teacher, the plan usually will fail. They should initially establish the best way to keep ongoing contact with the teacher, based on the instructional model that was selected. Should the consultant meet with the teacher weekly during a conference period or around school hours? Is the student in Content Mastery, requiring contact several times a week to coordinate supportive efforts? Has the student been placed in a Cooperative Learning structure with which the teacher is comfortable, requiring less ongoing contact?

However, regardless of the model, the teachers should meet at a predetermined time to consider if the new plan is successful. The mainstream teacher should be encouraged to observe student progress in learning and behavior on a daily basis to have data to discuss with the consultant. During evaluative meetings, the plan rarely needs to be discarded, even if the mainstream teacher seems discouraged and says "It just isn't working." At this point, the consultant should go back to the earlier steps, select which specific classroom requirements still are not being met, and modify the plan. Rarely does the baby need to be thrown out with the bath water; it is the support of the specialist that will keep the teacher from becoming discouraged.

Barbara asks, "But how can I have all these meetings with teachers when my direct contact hours with students increase annually? I won't have time to teach anyone."

As students begin to succeed in the mainstream classes, frequent conferences with teachers concerning all students may not be necessary, but there should be a monitoring system that allows the specialist to track student progress. Teachers in Carrollton-Farmers ISD have developed a checklist that is easy for mainstream teachers to complete, and that allows the Content Mastery teacher to have follow-up information and to be sure that problems are identified early. An adaptation of this form appears in Figure 6-1. The specialist sends a copy to the mainstream teacher, listing the names of all students enrolled in Content Mastery from any of the teacher's classes. It is important to note that not only are grades considered as criteria for success, but also behavior, homework completion, and problems in taking exams. This type of checklist also can be used by resource teachers or by specialists in the collaborative model discussed earlier. When a problem is indicated on the sheet, the specialist should meet with the mainstream teacher to discuss ways of improving the performance of the student. Since the teacher has indicated the existence of the problem to the specialist, a request for assistance usually can be understood.

Guidelines for Working with Other Professionals

Following are some general rules which may underscore successful interactions with educators in your school and district.

1. A student's failure in academics or inability to meet behavioral expectations can come from a variety of sources. Avoid blaming the mainstream teacher, parents, or other supportive staff who have worked with the student.

2. Accept the shift from the traditional expectation that you alone are responsible for the student's success. When speaking with other professionals, become part of a team, supporting their efforts and acting as a consultant.

3. Always make administrators aware of your efforts. While most teachers wait until there is a problem, administrators like hearing about the successful experiences and need to understand the special educational model you are using. They often feel awkward if they receive calls from parents and cannot respond because they are not knowledgeable about what you are doing. Administrators can be your best supporters if you include them in the excitement of your program. Subsequently, they will encourage teachers in the school to work with you cooperatively if they feel you can offer effective change strategies.

4. Accept that your way is not the only way when you are consulting with other educators. While your experiences may point you in one direction, try to be open-minded and flexible, understanding that the student likely behaves differently in other educational settings than in your room, and that a different type of strategy may be necessary. You can be an expert by working with teachers to suggest modifications, but you cannot always have the final say. The most important oucome is a successful experience for the mainstream teacher and the student.

5. Change takes time. Be patient, but give ongoing support to the teacher as your student action plan is implemented.

6. If the regular educator refuses to implement the plan you suggest, you may have to develop a new plan. The negative interactions caused by your insistence that the teacher adopt a particular strategy may damage your future ability to work not only with this teacher but with others in the building.

7. Whenever possible, suggest ideas that can be useful to more than one student in the mainstream so that additional students in the class can benefit.

8. Refuse to be a tutor. Your job is to help students overcome or compensate for their learning problems, not just to help them "get by" in general education, a situation that might otherwise always require supportive tutoring without any demonstration of real improvement in skills. However, instead of seeming negative in this refusal, you might offer to work with the teacher to remediate skill areas that are preventing the student from learning in the mainstream class.

Content Mastery Center Grade Check

Please check any or all of the pertinent items below. You may indicate student's grade by a number average or by checking the Maintaining 80 Average column. If this grade is not an 80 and failing, please check the failing Column also. I will conference with any student experiencing difficulty. Any student not maintaining an 80 average must use the Center. Thanks for all your effort and support.

Teacher_____ Course_____ Dates: From _____ to _____

STUDENT UPDATE CHECKLIST | MAINTAINING 80 AVERAGE

Students	Period	Average	Yes	No	Failing	Behavior Problems	Homework Problems	Test Problems	Other

Figure 6-1. Content Mastery Center Grade Check. Reprinted with permission, Carrollton-Farmers Branch ISD, Texas.

9. Work closely, not only with mainstream teachers, but also with other specialists involved with the student. Since learning disabilities include such an array of areas, specialists will be in varied fields, such as reading, speech, psychology, counseling, neurology, and school nursing. If the home has become dysfunctional, other professionals such as social workers and representatives of the courts may be involved. When working with other specialists it is critical to clarify responsibilities, both to eliminate conflicts and avoid overlap or gaps in functions (Lerner, 1988).

10. Be part of a team providing in-service training in learning disabilities for teachers, administrators, teaching assistants, and other specialists. Throughout training activities, emphasize specific methods and materials for successfully integrating students into general education. You might under-score your own availability for consultation and support.

WORKING WITH PARENTS

Unfortunately, in many situations involving parents of students with learning disabilities, there is an uneasy peace, or no peace at all with the teacher. "So true," notes Barbara. "With many parents it seems as if we are on opposite sides of a fence with the child in the middle. I can't help feeling critical when parents are angry at *me* over their child's difficulties at school, and I'm the one who spends my day, and night, worrying over how to improve the situation. Then there are the parents who never return calls, don't come to open houses, and just don't seem to care. Sometimes dealing with the child is a lot easier than dealing with the parents."

Once again, Barbara is describing the perceptions of many teachers based on their daily frustrations. However, there is more to the story than appearances. As Lerner (1988) notes, research on mothers' attitudes toward their children who are handicapped indicates several common patterns. Some reject and criticize the child's behavior, with a resultant lowering of child self-esteem. These children rarely tend to feel successful and may not even attempt tasks difficult for them because of a lack of encouragement internalized into a feeling of helplessness. Another mother-child relationship may result in overcompensation for the child's handicap. Parents may make the child the center of their life and family. Training may be overly zealous and expectations too high. These families may blame the school when their goals for the child are not reached, usually faulting the teacher or special education program. According to the research, another type of mother accepts the child and the handicap, is able to carry on a normal life, giving support to the child, but not negating other family needs. This type of parent tends to be the most supportive of special educators.

Parental reactions also strongly depend on when the handicap is identified: this may be at birth or an early age for the more severely handicapped, but not until years later for a child with a less immediately noticed handicap such as a learning disability. If the problem first is discussed at a school placement meeting, professionals have to be prepared to face stages of denial, anger, and the subsequent seeking of additional diagnoses on the part of the parent. These feelings are real and often very strong, but should be anticipated. This is not a time for educators to become subjective and to believe that negative comments are directed toward them personally, but to understand how they would feel if they had just learned that their child had a serious problem that might affect their future. Parents have different needs at different stages of dealing with their child's problem. Parents of younger students or those who have newly learned of the problem will tend to be more upset and angry than those who have dealt with the problem over a longer period of time, have learned to better understand their child and the educational system.

Guidelines for Working with Parents

As in working with other professionals, there are a series of guidelines to support interactions with parents, from daily routines to individual conferences.

1. In your school and district, develop support groups for parents of students with learning disabilities. There is no better way for parents to accept their child's learning differences than to share their feelings with others experiencing the same thing. Parents respond best to other parents, making it imperative that the group be conducted by members, not by teachers. But the school and district can help organize groups by contacting the most involved parents to lead the effort, providing a place for meetings, and clerical support to mail out announcements. While some of the meetings might be parents getting to know each other and sharing their methods of dealing with home- and school-related problems, others could be presentations by parents or specialists on critical topics, such as social skills development, discipline, language development, or vocational opportunities. Educators could attend these meetings when invited to demonstrate support and share programming information. Parents also should be encouraged to join groups such as the Association for Children and Adults with Learning Disabilities, an organization that has been powerful in expanding services and which helps parents become involved in advocacy programs.

2. It is often sad to learn that even after years of special education placement for their child, many parents do not understand the nature of the learning disability. When something is not understood, it can become threatening or at least leave parents with feelings of uncertainty about what to do and what the disability will mean for the child's adulthood. Parents who understand that their child has difficulty comprehending conversation or directions can modify the home environment and adjust their own expectations more easily than parents who have been told that their child has "receptive aphasia." Whether in the initial placement meeting or when informally discussing students' difficulties and progress, specialists should *never use technical language.* Parents should be encouraged to ask questions and to call upon specialists to interpret why their child may be behaving in a particular manner. The teacher of students with learning disabilities can serve as a consultant to parents as well as to other educators. Once parents understand their child's problems and are offered productive ways of managing the child, the student begins to succeed more quickly.

3. Make contact early in the year to introduce yourself to parents and to communicate your interest in their child. A new resource teacher who had taken over a difficult teaching assignment midyear found herself rejected both by parents and students. They finally had become attached to the previous teacher who subsequently had moved to another community. No one seemed willing to go through the effort of getting to know the new teacher or to even accept that she could be successful. Despite numerous other tasks attached to the new job, during her first 2 weeks on campus, she called the parents

of every child, expressing her pleasure at having the child in her class and discussing her teaching policies with the parents. To the parents she could not reach, she personally mailed an introductory letter, describing her background and her excitement at her new job. Within the first month, the principal was stopped by several parents excited by the teacher's enthusiasm. She had developed her own strong support group who now viewed her as capable of being highly successful.

4. Most parents do want to know what is going on in their child's classroom and enjoy receiving communications from teachers. The classroom program can be described through open houses and newsletters sent home, the latter often including a chatty discussion of individual student successes as well as a more general overview of curriculum. An informed parent is rarely a critical one, especially if the teacher shows a caring attitude toward the students.

5. Many parents want to know what they can do at home to improve their child's learning. Yet, it is rarely a good idea to encourage parents to work with their children on academic tasks: the parents tend to become frustrated and the children experience failure in front of the most significant adults in their life (Lerner, 1988). Instead of having parents work on academic tasks, it often is best to suggest that they model and guide their children in the development of social and independent living skills, from politeness during conversation to budgeting and driving. It also is important to encourage them to take time to enjoy their children, doing nothing instructional at all, just leisure activities for the whole family. Family time tends to take away the focus of parents on any specific child and lets the children know there is more to life, and their self-esteem, than schoolwork.

6. An adjunct to this is to not ask the parents to do more than their time allowance or family pressures will allow. For example, parents might be asked to support their child's homework performance by having a quiet place for the student to work and a designated hour and by checking to be sure that everything on the assignment sheet has been completed. But they should not be expected to spend every evening at the child's elbow teaching the assignment. With so many single-parent families and pressured work schedules, teachers must not expect parents to spend large amounts of instructional time with children during evenings and weekends.

7. When parents are working at home to assist their child's school performance, a note or phone call from the teacher acknowledging the support always is wonderful reinforcement.

8. The Parent Center for the Albuquerque Public Schools points out that during conferences with parents, it is best to begin and end on a positive note, setting the tone for the meeting. Teachers should share positive information before attempting to solve problems. They note that it is critical to listen and to encourage sharing so that parents will know that their ideas are respected.

9. Teachers should send positive notes home with students, noting successes or even attempts at work previously refused. It is not surprising that even the most disorganized students rarely lose these messages. The notes also give students an opportunity to discuss their schoolwork with parents and for the family to provide positive reinforcement.

10. Parents should be invited to observe in the classroom during designated periods. While parents would disrupt the class by wandering in and out during unscheduled times, inviting parents, grandparents, and siblings to visit during special activities allows everyone to become more comfortable with the school environment and with your room in particular.

11. Communicate with parents when you are observing a small problem starting to escalate. Content Mastery teachers in Carrollton-Farmers use the form in Figure 6-2 to monitor student behaviors across classes, then sharing the information with parents. Use of this system informs the student that teachers and parents together are concerned about school behavior. Prevention is much more powerful than later reaction to a major problem. If a conference is held, when initiating discussion of the developing problem, it is best to use terms like "we" ("What can we do?" or "How can we best work together?") to show parents that you are working with them and that a team approach to a solution may be best. Be careful not to criticize the child, but to deal more objectively with the developing problem.

12. Ask parents the most difficult problem they are experiencing with the student at home and, if possible, work together to solve it. Maria was a very quiet, well-mannered middle school student who had grown attached to her special education teacher and was cooperative and eager to please. Yet, during a conversation with the teacher, the mother shared that Maria was a tyrant at home in the morning, disturbing the routine of the entire family and sending everyone off angry and exhausted. She hated to get out of bed, needing numerous calls, then made negative comments to everyone around her, and often made her parents late to work.

The teacher explored Maria's bedtime with the mother and found that she was allowed to stay up as late as her older brothers and sisters, two of whom were out of school and working. Since she was much more pleasant in the evening, the family enjoyed her company and failed to realize that they were aiding her morning disposition through a late bedtime. The teacher suggested the bedtime change, but also noted that she would like to help since she had a good rapport with the student. With Maria sharing in the conversation, the teacher asked the mother to buy a clock radio and allow Maria to set it for as much time as she needed in the morning. Since Maria was "becoming an adult," the teacher suggested that she might be left alone to get herself ready for school; if she took too long, she would have to miss breakfast. Her parents were instructed to leave at a certain hour for work and to have her walk to school if she were not ready to go, suffering an afternoon detention if she were late. The mother was asked to send a note with her daily for the teacher, simply stating if the morning went well or poorly. With a hug, the teacher told Maria that she would look forward to seeing the note each morning before she attended classes, and that she would allow Maria a special privilege, such as passing out materials, each day that the note was positive.

The outcome was immediately effective. Maria wanted to please the teacher and was delighted at her new adult status at home, willing to trade the later bedtime on school nights for the positive attention she received from parents and siblings. A rare happening: She never brought a negative note, and after the first few weeks told the teacher that she really did not need the extra activities. Her real reward was visiting with the teacher each morning.

Later that year, the teacher was given a check for $100 from the school PTA. Maria's mother was PTA secretary and had noted in her classroom visits that more materials were needed to support students in special education. She had initiated a

PARENT'S SIGNATURE _____

Content Mastery Daily Check List

Please check the appropriate boxes for this student's performance today. Thanks!

Name _____   Date _____

Course	Teacher's Signature	Behavior Approp. Inapp.		Arrived On Time Yes No		Materials All Some None			On Task Yes No		Classwork Yes No		Attempted Homework Yes No N/A		

The student will have a conference with the CM teacher reviewing this form at the end of the day.

Figure 6-2. Content Mastery Daily Check List. Reprinted with permission, Carrollton-Farmers Branch ISD, Texas.

discussion with PTA members, underscoring how excellent the teacher was, and they had agreed. It was her way of saying "Thank you." Parents appreciate help for their children.

SUMMARY

This chapter included ways of developing cooperation between the learning disabilities specialist, other professionals, and parents. In working with professionals, it is viewed as necessary to encourage a philosophical shift from isolation to integration, where educators work together in teams to determine ways of teaching students who learn differently.

One method explored was the Mainstream Assistance Team (Fuchs & Fuchs, 1989), a consultation model where special and regular educators work together in a prereferral stage when developing problems first are indicated. The learning specialist serves as an invaluable team member who observes students' classroom behavior, suggests intervention strategies, and provides follow-up materials and support.

Additionally, the Consulting Teacher model was viewed as invaluable once students are enrolled in special education. A series of steps were listed to allow specialists to work with mainstream teachers cooperatively, gauging what requirements the student has not been able to meet and developing appropriate methods for future teaching. The specialist was advised to understand the teacher's situation as clearly as possible in order to be empathetic, and to be realistic in expectations about changes the teacher would be willing to make and the student to accept.

A number of guidelines were discussed which can provide a framework for successful interactions with other educators. From avoiding blame to providing ideas that can work with a variety of students in the mainstream class, the specialist serves not only as a team member, but also as an agent of change.

Ways of working with parents were reviewed next. The special educator was asked to understand parents' perspective. Some parents may reject the child who is handicapped, resulting in much criticism and a subsequent lowering of the child's self-esteem. Others may attempt to overly compensate for the handicap, making the child the center of their family, adopting a zealous attitude and unrealistic expectations. The third pattern is acceptance, where the family unit functions normally and the parents are able to deal with the handicap. Teachers should be aware of the way individual parents feel and the type of expectations they have for child behavior. They also should be alert to the amount of time the family has had to deal with the learning difference so that they can be as supportive as the parents' needs indicate.

Guidelines were suggested to establish positive interactions with parents. The development of support groups where parents share their experiences with others in similar situations may be critical to full acceptance of the child's problems and awareness of sound programming options for the future. Helping parents understand the nature of the learning difference and the ways the program will affect change also is imperative, based on the use of nontechnical language in discussions and the need for ongoing communication from teachers.

The philosophy educators are encouraged to adopt is one that has underscored all the chapters in this book: Teachers need to take charge of classroom interactions with students, be involved in collaboration with other educators, and establish a cooperative attitude with parents. Instead of the isolation that has traditionally plagued, and more recently defeated, many special education programs, the teacher and student have to become participants in the larger school community where their needs are viewed as equally important to those of other teachers and students. It's not so overwhelming, Barbara, if you're not alone.

REFERENCES

American Psychiatric Association (1987). *Diagnostic and statistical manual of mental disorders* (3rd ed.). Washington, DC: American Psychiatric Association.

Axelrod, S. (1977). *Behavior modification for the classroom teacher.* New York: McGraw-Hill.

Barsch, R. (1965). Six factors in learning. In J. Helmuth (Ed.), *Learning Disorders* (Vol.1). Seattle: Special Child Publications.

Berliner, D.C. (1984). The half-full glass: A review of research on teaching. In P.L. Hosford (Ed.), *Using what we know about teaching* (pp. 51-77). Alexandria, VA: Association for Supervision and Curriculum Development.

Bickel, W., & Bickel, D. (1986). Effective schools, classrooms and instruction: Implications for special education. *Exceptional Children, 20*(6), 489-519.

Brophy, J., & Good, T. (1986). Teaching behavior and student achievement. In M. Wittock (Ed.), *Handbook of research and teaching* (3rd ed., pp. 328-375). New York: Macmillan.

Canter, L. (1976). *Assertive discipline: A take-charge approach for today's educator.* Seal Beach, CA: Canter and Associates.

Charles, C.M. (1989). *Building classroom discipline* (3rd ed). New York: Longman.

Cosden, M., & Semmel, M. (1987). Developmental changes in micro-educational environments for learning handicapped and non-learning handicapped elementary school students. *Journal of Special Education Technology, 3*(4), 1-13.

Davis, L.C. (1989). Collaboration and collegiality among regular and special educators: Restructuring to meet the needs of students at risk. Unpublished paper prepared for meeting course requirements, Trinity University, San Antonio, TX.

Elkind, D. (1988). *The hurried child.* Reading, MA: Addison-Wesley.

Elkind, D. (1989). *All grown up and no place to go.* Reading, MA: Addison-Wesley.

Fuchs, D., & Fuchs, L.S. (1989). Exploring effective and efficient prereferral interventions: A component analysis of Behavioral Consultation. *School Psychology Review, 18,* 260-283.

Fuchs, D., Fuchs, L., Gilman, S., Reeder, P., Bahr, M. Fernstrom, P., & Roberts, H. (1990). Prefeferral intervention through teacher consultation: Mainstream assistance teams. *Academic Therapy, 25*(3), 263-276.

Gallagher, J. (1991). *Special education for the future.* Paper presented at the meeting of the Trinity University Education Lecture Series, San Antonio, TX.

Ginott, H. (1971). *Teacher and child.* New York: Macmillan.

Gottlieb, J. (1982). Mainstreaming: Fulfilling the promise? *American Journal of Mental Deficiency, 86,* 115-126.

Hewett, F. (1968). *The emotionally disturbed child in the classroom.* Boston: Allyn and Bacon.

Hunter, M. (1984). Knowing, teaching and supervising. In P.L. Hosford (Ed.), *What we know about teaching* (pp. 169-192). Alexandria, VA: Association for Supervision and Curriculum Development.

Idol, L., West, J.F., & Lloyd, S.R.(1988). Organizing and implementing specialized reading programs: A collaborative approach involving classroom, remedial, and special education teachers. *Remedial and Special Education, 9* (2), 54-61.

Johnson, D., Johnson, R., & Holubec, E.J. (1986). *Circles of learning.* Edina, MN: Interaction Book Company.

Jones, F. (1987). *Positive classroom discipline.* New York: McGraw-Hill.

Kirk, S. (1963). Behavioral diagnosis and remediation of learning disabilities. In *Conference on the exploration into the problems of the perceptually handicapped child.* Evanston, IL: Fund for the Perceptually Handicapped Child.

Kounin, J. (1977). *Discipline and group management in classrooms.* New York: Holt, Rinehart and Winston

Ladoucer, R., & Armstrong, J. (1983). Evaluation of a behavioral program for the improvement of grades among high school students. *Journal of Counseling Psychology, 30,* 100-103.

Laurie, T., Buchwach, L., Silverman, R., & Zigmond, N. (1978). Teaching secondary learning disabled students in the mainstream. *Learning Disabilities Quarterly, 1,* 62-71.

Lerner, J. (1988). *Learning disabilities: Theories, diagnosis, and teaching strategies* (5th ed.). Dallas: Houghton Mifflin.

Mandell, C., & Gold, V. (1984). *Teaching handicapped students.* St. Paul, MN: West Publishing.

Moran, M.R. (1978). *Assessment of the exceptional learner in the regular classroom.* Denver, CO: Love.

Morsink, C., Soar, S., Soar, R., & Thomas, R. (1986). Research on teaching: Opening the door to special education classrooms. *Exceptional Children, 53*(1), 32-40.

Redl, F., & Wattenberg, W. (1951). *Mental hygiene in teaching.* New York: Harcourt, Brace and World.

Reynolds, M.C., & Birch, J.W. (1988). *Adaptive mainstreaming: A primer for teachers and principals* (3rd ed.). New York: Longman.

Rosenshine, B., & Stevens, R. (1986). Teaching functions. In M. Wittrock (Ed.), *Handbook of research on teaching* (3rd ed., pp. 376-391). New York: Macmillan.

Sharpley, C. (1985). Implicit rewards in the classroom. *Contemporary Educational Psychology, 10,* 349-368.

Skinner, B.F. (1971). *Beyond freedom and dignity.* New York: Knopf.

Slavin, R.E. (1983). *Cooperative learning.* New York: Longman.

Smith, S. (1981). *No easy answers: The learning disabled child at home and at school.* New York: Bantam Books.

Waldron, K.A. (1985). The effects of an intermediary placement on learning-disabled and low-achieving adolescents. *The Journal of Learning Disabilities, 18*(3), 154-159.

Waldron, K.A., & Saphire, D.G. (1990). An analysis of WISC-R factors for learning-disabled/gifted students. *The Journal of Learning Disabilities, 23*(8), 491-498.

Wang, M.C., & Birch, J.W. (1984). Effective special education in regular classes. *Exceptional Children, 53,* 77-79.

SUBJECT INDEX